CW00586407

KETO DIET FOR WOMEN

This Book Includes : "Keto Diet For Women Over 50 + Keto For Women Over 50 "

By Jason Smith

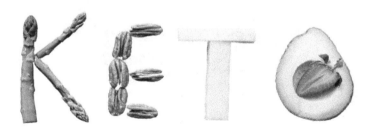

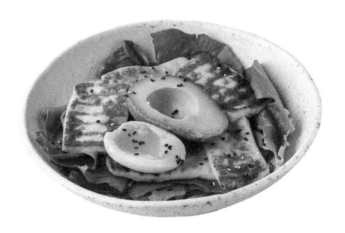

© **Copyright 2021 by (Jason Smith) - all rights reserved.**

This document is geared towards providing exact and reliable information in regards to the topic and issue covered. The publication is sold with the idea that the publisher is not required to render accounting, officially permitted, or otherwise, qualified services. If advice is necessary, legal or professional, a practiced individual in the profession should be ordered.

- From a declaration of principles which was accepted and approved equally by a committee of the American bar association and a committee of publishers and associations.

In no way is it legal to reproduce, duplicate, or transmit any part of this document in either electronic means or printed format. Recording of this publication is strictly prohibited, and any storage of this document is not allowed unless with written permission from the publisher. All rights reserved.

The information provided herein is stated to be truthful and consistent, in that any liability, in terms of inattention or otherwise, by any usage or abuse of any policies, processes, or directions contained within is the solitary and utter responsibility of the recipient reader. Under no circumstances will any legal responsibility or blame be held against the publisher for reparation, damages, or monetary loss due to the information herein, either directly or indirectly.

Respective authors own all copyrights not held by the publisher.

The information herein is offered for informational purposes solely and is universal as such. The presentation of the information is without a contract or any type of guarantee assurance.

The trademarks used are without any consent, and the publication of the trademark is without permission or backing by the trademark owner. All trademarks and brands within this book are for clarifying purposes only and are owned by the owners themselves, not affiliated with this document.

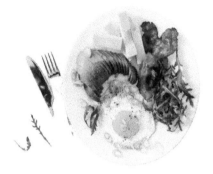

KETO DIET FOR WOMEN OVER 50

Contents

Table of contents

KETO FOR WOMEN OVER 50

Conclusion 211

KETO DIET FOR WOMEN OVER 50

The Complete Ketogenic Diet Step by Step To Learn How to Easily Lose Weight for Woman

By Jason Smith

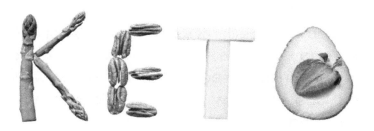

Introduction

The keto diet is a diet that has higher and lower fat values. It decreases glucose & insulin levels and changes the body's digestion away from carbohydrates and more towards fat & ketones. A word used in a low-carb diet is "Ketogenic." The concept is to provide more calories from fat and protein and few from sugars. The consumption of a high, low-sugar diet, adequate-protein, is used in medicine to achieve difficult (unstable) epilepsy control in young people. Instead of sugar, the diet allows the body to eat fats. Usually, the nutritious starches are converted to sugar, which will then be distributed throughout the body and is particularly important in filling the mind's work. Keto diet can cause enormous declines in the levels of glucose and insulin.

How food affects your body

Our metabolic procedures survive if we do not get the right details, and our well-being declines. We can get overweight, malnourished, and at risk for the worsening of diseases and disorders, such as inflammatory disease, diabetes, and cardiovascular disease if women get an unhealthy amount of essential nutrients or nourishment that provides their body with inadequate guidance. The dietary supplements allow the cells in our bodies to serve their essential capacities. This quote from a well-known workbook shows how dietary supplements are important for our physical work. Supplements are the nourishment feed substances necessary for the growth, development, and support of the body's capacities. Fundamental claimed that when a supplement is absent, capability sections and thus decrease in human health. The metabolic processes are delayed when the intake of supplements usually may not fulfill the cell activity's supplement requirements.

The keto diet involves keeping to a relatively low-carb, high-fat diet to put the body into a physiological state called ketosis. This makes fat intake increasingly productive for the health. When starting the diet, the ketogenic diet can induce a decrease in the drive, as the dieter will suffer side effects of carb removal and possibly low carb influenza. Whenever the detox and influenza-like symptoms have gone, and the dieter has transitioned to the reduced way of living, leading to weight loss from the diet, the charisma would in all likelihood reset and probably be comparable to earlier. Although the drive alert has a lot of credibility in the mainstream, in other words, supplementation provides advice to our bodies on how to function. In this sense, nourishment can be seen as a source of "information for the body." Pondering food along these lines gives one a view of the nourishment beyond calories or grams, fantastic food sources, or bad food sources. Instead of avoiding food sources, this perspective pushes us to reflect on the nutrients we can add. Instead of reviewing nourishment as the enemy, we look at nourishment to reduce health and disease by having the body look after ability.

Kidney and Heart Disease

When the body is low in electrolytes and fluid over the increased pee, electrolyte loss, such as magnesium, sodium, and potassium, can be caused. This will render people inclined to suffer serious kidney problems. Flushing out is not a joke and can lead to light-headedness, damage to the kidney, or kidney problems. Just like electrolytes are essential for the heart's standard stomping, this can place a dieter at the risk of cardiac arrhythmia. "Electrolyte appears to lack are not joking, and that may bring in an irregular heartbeat, that can be harmful,"

Yo-yo Dieting designs

When individuals encounter difficulties staying on the prohibitive diet indefinitely, the keto diet will also cause yo-yo dieting. That can have other adverse effects on the body.

Other effects

Other responses can involve terrible breath, fatigue, obstruction, irregular menstrual periods, reduced bone density, and trouble with rest. For even the most part, other consequences are not so much considered since it is impossible to observe dieters on a long-term assumption to discover the food schedule's permanent effects.

Wholesome Concerns

"There is still a dread amongst healthcare professionals that certain high intakes of extremely unhealthy fats will have a longer journey negative effect," she explained. Weight loss will also, for the time being, complicate the data. As overweight people get in form, paying less attention to how they do so, they sometimes end up with much better lipid profiles and blood glucose levels.

In comparison, the keto diet is extremely low in particular natural ingredients, fruits, nuts, and veggies that are as nutritious as a whole. Without these supplements, fiber, some carbohydrates, minerals, including phytochemicals that come along with these nourishments, will move through people on a diet. In the long run, this has vital public health consequences, such as bone degradation and increased risk of infinite diseases.

Sodium

The mixture of sodium (salt), fat, sugar, including bunches of sodium, will make inexpensive food more delicious for many people. However, diets rich in sodium will trigger fluid retention, which is why you can feel puffy, bloated, or swelled up in the aftermath of consuming cheap food. For those with pulse problems, a diet rich in sodium is also harmful. Sodium can increase circulatory stress and add weight to the cardiovascular structure. If one survey reveals, about % of grown-ups lose how much salt is in their affordable food meals. The study looked at 993 adults and found that the initial prediction was often smaller than the actual figure (1,292 mg). This suggests the sodium gauges in the abundance of 1,000 mg is off. One affordable meal could be worth a significant proportion of your day.

Impact on the Respiratory Framework

An overabundance of calories can contribute to weight gain from cheap foods. This will add to the weight. Obesity creates the risk of respiratory conditions, including asthma with shortness of breath. The extra pounds can put pressure on the heart and lungs, and with little intervention, side effects can occur. When you walk, climb stairs, or work out, you can notice trouble breathing. For youngsters, the possibility of respiratory problems is especially obvious. One research showed that young people who consume cheap food at least three days a week are bound to develop asthma.

Impact on the focal sensory system

For the time being, cheap food may satisfy hunger; however, long-haul effects are more detrimental. Individuals who consume inexpensive food and processed bakery items are 51 percent bound to generate depression than people who do not eat or eat either of those foods.

Impact on the conceptive framework

The fixings in cheap food and lousy nourishment can affect your money. One analysis showed that phthalates are present in prepared nourishment. Phthalates are synthetic compounds that can mess with the way your body's hormones function. Introduction to substantial amounts of these synthetics, like birth absconds, could prompt regenerative problems.

Impact on the integumentary framework (skin, hair, nails)

The food you eat may affect your skin's appearance, but it's not going to be the food you imagine. The responsibility for skin dry out breakouts has traditionally been claimed by sweets and sticky nourishments such as pizza. Nevertheless, as per the Mayo Clinic, there are starches. Carb-rich foods cause glucose jumps, and these sudden leaps in glucose levels can induce inflammation of the skin. Additionally, as shown by one investigation, young people and young women who consume inexpensive food at any pace three days a week are expected to create skin inflammation. Dermatitis is a skin disease that causes dry, irritated skin spots that are exacerbated.

Impact on the skeletal framework (bones)

Acids in the mouth can be enlarged by carbohydrates and sugar in inexpensive food and treated food. These acids may distinguish tooth lacquer. Microorganisms can take hold when the tooth veneer disappears, and depressions can occur. Weight will also prompt issues with bone thickness and bulk. The more severe chance of falling and breaking bones is for heavy individuals. It is important to continue training, develop muscles that support the bones, and sustain a balanced diet to prevent bone loss. One investigation showed that the measure of calories, sugar, and sodium in cheap food meals remains, to a large degree, constant because of attempts to bring problems to light and make women more intelligent consumers. As women get busier and eat out more often, it could have antagonistic effects on women and America's healthcare structure.

Chapter 1: Keto Diet and Its Benefits

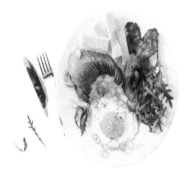

In the case of a ketogenic diet, the aim is to restrict carbohydrate intake to break down fat for power. When this occurs, to produce ketones that are by-products of the metabolism, the liver breaks down fat. These ketones are used in the absence of glucose to heat the body. A ketogenic diet takes the body into a "ketosis" mode. A metabolic condition that happens as ketone bodies in the blood contains most of the body's energy rather than glucose from carbohydrate-produced foods (such as grains, all sources of sugar or fruit). This compares with a glycolytic disorder, where blood glucose produces most of the body's power.

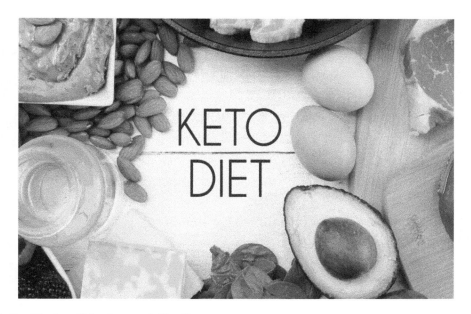

1.1. Keto Diet and its Success

The keto diet is successful in many studies, especially among obese men and women. The results suggest that KD can help manage situations such as:

- Obesity.

- Heart disease.

It is difficult to relate the ketogenic diet to cardiovascular disease risk factors. Several studies have shown that keto diets may contribute to substantial reductions in overall cholesterol, rises in levels of HDL cholesterol, decreases in levels of triglycerides and decreases in levels of LDL cholesterol, as well as possible changes in levels of blood pressure.

- Neurological disorders, including Alzheimer's, dementia, multiple sclerosis and Parkinson's.

- Polycystic ovarian syndrome (PCOS), among women of reproductive age, is the most prevalent endocrine condition.
- Certain forms of cancer, including cancers of the liver, colon, pancreas and ovaries.
- Diabetes Type 2. Among type 2 diabetics, it can also minimize the need for drugs.
- Seizure symptoms and seizures.
- And others.

•

1.2. Why Do the Ketogenic Diet

By exhausting the body from its sugar store, Ketogenic works to start sorting fat and protein for vitality, inducing ketosis (and weight loss).

1. Helps in weight loss

To convert fat into vitality, it takes more effort than it takes to turn carbohydrates into vitality. A ketogenic diet along these lines can help speed up weight loss. In comparison, because the diet is rich in protein, it doesn't leave you starving as most diets do. Five findings uncovered tremendous weight loss from a ketogenic diet in a meta-examination of 13 complex randomized controlled preliminaries.

2. Diminishes skin break out

There are different causes for the breakout of the skin, and food and glucose can be established. Eating a balanced diet of prepared and refined sugars can alter gut microorganisms and emphasize sensational variances in glucose, both of which would affect the skin's health. Therefore, that is anything but surprising that a keto diet may reduce a few instances of skin inflammation by decreasing carb entry.

3. May help diminish the danger of malignancy

There has been a lot of study on the ketogenic diet and how it could effectively forestall or even cure those malignant growths. One investigation showed that the ketogenic diet might be a corresponding effective treatment with chemotherapy and radiation in people with malignancy. It is because it can cause more oxidative concern than in ordinary cells in malignancy cells.

Some hypotheses indicate that it may decrease insulin entanglements, which could be linked to some cancers because the ketogenic diet lowers elevated glucose.

4. Improves heart health

There is some indication that the diet will boost cardiac health by lowering cholesterol by accessing the ketogenic diet in a balanced manner (which looks at avocados as a healthy fat rather than pork skins). One research showed that LDL ("Terrible") cholesterol levels fundamentally expanded among those adopting the keto diet. In turn, the LDL ("terrible") cholesterol fell.

5. May secure mind working

More study into the ketogenic diet and even the mind is needed. A few studies indicate that the keto diet has Neuro-protective effects. These can help treat or curtail Parkinson's, Alzheimer's, and even some rest problems. One research also showed that young people had increased and psychological work during a ketogenic diet.

6. Possibly lessens seizures

The theory that the combination of fat, protein, and carbohydrates modifies how vitality is utilized by the body, inducing ketosis. Ketosis is an abnormal level of Ketone in the blood. In people with epilepsy, ketosis will prompt a reduction in seizures.

7. Improves health in women with PCOS

An endocrine condition that induces augmented ovaries with pimples is polycystic ovarian disorder PCOS). On the opposite, a high-sugar diet can affect those with PCOS. On the ketogenic diet and PCOS, there are not many clinical tests. One pilot study involving five women on 24 weeks showed that the ketogenic diet:

- Aided hormone balance
- Improved luteinizing hormone (ILH)/follicle-invigorating hormone (FSH) proportions
- Increased weight loss
- Improved fasting insulin

For children who suffer the adverse effects of a particular problem (such as Lennox-gastaut disease or Rett disorder) and do not respond to seizure prescription, keto is also prescribed as suggested by the epilepsy foundation.

They note that the number of seizures these children had can be greatly reduced by keto, with 10 to 15 percent turns out to be sans seizure. It may also help patients to reduce the portion of their prescription in some circumstances. Be it as it can, the ketogenic diet still many effective trials to back up its advantages. For adults with epilepsy, the keto diet can likewise be helpful. It was considered as preferable to other diets in supporting people with:

- Epilepsy
- Type 2 diabetes
- Type 1 diabetes
- High blood pressure
- Heart disease
- Polycystic ovary syndrome
- Fatty liver disease
- Cancer
- Migraines

25

- Alzheimer's infection
- Parkinson's infection
- Chronic inflammation
- High blood sugar levels
- Obesity

The ketogenic diet will be beneficial, regardless of whether you are not in danger from any of these disorders. A portion of the advantages that are enjoyed by the vast majority are:

- An increment in vitality
- Improved body arrangement
- Better cerebrum work
- A decline in aggravation

As should be clear, the ketogenic diet has a vast variety of advantages, but is it preferable to other diets?

8. Treating epilepsy — the origins of the ketogenic diet

Until sometime in 1998, the major analysis on epilepsy and the keto diets was not distributed. Of about 150 children, almost each of whom had several seizures a week, despite taking two psychosis drugs in either situation. The children were given a one-year initial ketogenic diet. Around 34 percent of infants, or slightly more than 33 percent, had a 90 percent decline in seizures after three months.

The healthy diet was claimed to be "more feasible than just a substantial lot of new anticonvulsant medications and is much endured by families and kids when it is effective." Not only was the keto diet supportive. It was, however, more useful than other drugs usually used.

9. Improving blood pressure with the ketogenic diet

A low-sugar intake is more effective at reducing the pulse than just a low-fat or moderate-fat diet. Restricting starches often provides preferable results over the mix of a low-fat regimen and a relaxing weight-loss/pulse.

10. The power to improve Alzheimer's disease

Alzheimer's disease patients also agree with organic chemistry." high sugar acceptance deepens academic performance in patient populations with Alzheimer's infectious disease." It means that more starches are consumed in the cerebrum. Will the reverse (trying to eat fewer carbs) improve the functioning of the cerebrum?

Other mental health benefits that ketone bodies have:

- They forestall neuronal loss.
- They ensure synapses against various sorts of damage.
- They save neuron work.

•

1.3. The Benefits of Ketogenic Diet

The board provides many substantial advantages when choosing a ketogenic diet for diabetes. Living in a stable ketosis state causes a tremendous change in blood glucose regulation and weight loss. Other frequent advantages provided include:

- Improvements in insulin affectability
- Lower circulatory strain
- Usually enhancements in cholesterol levels.
- Reduced reliance on taking drugs

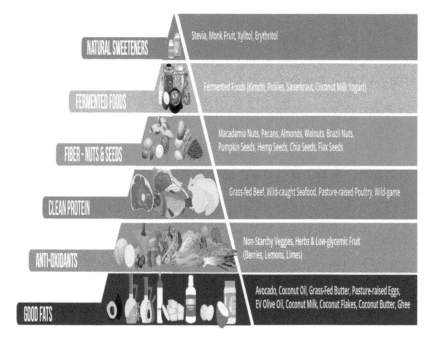

We send you a short science behind the ketogenic diet in this book and how it attempts to give these particular benefits.

1. Weight loss and support

The ketogenic diet's significant benefit is achieving accelerated weight loss, reducing starches necessary to be in a ketosis state, causing both a noteworthy decrease in muscle vs. fats and bulk increase and maintenance. Studies have shown that a low-carb, keto diet can produce an all-inclusive duration of solid weight loss. For one year, a big person had the opportunity to lose, by and large, 15 kilograms. It was 3 kg, which is more than the low-fat food used in the study carried out.

2. Blood glucose control

The other main reason for maintaining a ketogenic diet for people with diabetes is its ability to reduce and regulate glucose levels. The substitute (macronutrient) that improves glucose the most is starch. Since the keto diet is low in starch, the greater rises in glucose are dispensed with. Ketogenic diets prove that they are effective in reducing hba1c, a long-term blood glucose regulation percentage. A natural decrease of 17 mmol/mol (1.5 percent) in hba1c levels for persons with type 2 diabetes. People with other forms of diabetes, such as diabetes and LADA, can also expect to see a strong decline in glucose levels and increase control. Remember that if an increase in blood glucose regulation is sustained over different years, this will reduce intricacies. It is necessary to play it safe for those on insulin, or otherwise at risk of hypos, to avoid the incidence of hypos.

Decreasing drug reliance on diabetes. Since it is so effective at lowering glucose levels, the keto diet provides the added benefit of allowing people with type 2 diabetes to decrease their dependency on diabetes medication.

Persons on insulin and other hypertension prescriptions (Sulphonylureas & Glinides, for example) may need to reduce their portions before initiating a ketogenic diet to avoid hypotension. For advice on this, contact your primary care provider.

3. Insulin affectability

To further restore insulin affectability, a ketogenic diet has emerged since it dispenses with the root driver of insulin obstruction, which is too high insulin levels in the bloodstream. This diet advances supported periods with low insulin since low carbohydrate levels indicate lower insulin levels. A high diet of starch resembles putting petroleum on the insulin obstruction fire. A more influential need for insulin is indicated by elevated sugar, and this aggravates insulin opposition. A ketogenic diet, by correlation, turns down insulin levels since fat is the least insulin-requiring macronutrient. In comparison, bringing the insulin levels down also helps with fat intake, provided that elevated insulin levels inhibit fat breakdown. The body will differentiate fat cells at the point that insulin levels decrease for several hours.

4. Hypertension control

It is estimated that 16 million people in the U.K. suffer from hypertension. Hypertension, for example, cardiovascular disease, stroke, and renal disease, is related to the scope of health disorders. Different studies have demonstrated that a ketogenic diet can reduce circulatory stress levels in overweight or type 2 diabetes people. It is also a part of metabolic imbalance.

5. Cholesterol levels

For the most part, ketogenic diets bring in reductions in cholesterol levels. LDL cholesterol levels are usually reduced, and HDL cholesterol levels increase, which is healthy. The amount of absolute cholesterol to HDL is possibly the most substantiated proportion of safe cholesterol. It can be effectively detected by taking the full cholesterol result and partitioning it by your HDLS result. It indicates good cholesterol, on the off chance that the amount you get is 3.5 or lower. Study findings suggest that ketogenic diets are normally possible to increase this proportion of good cholesterol.

After starting a ketogenic, a few individuals can display an expansion in LDL and all-out cholesterol. It is generally taken as a bad indicator, but this does not speak of compounding in heart health if the absolute cholesterol to HDL ratio is appropriate.

Cholesterol is a confounding topic, and if your cholesterol levels essentially shift on a ketogenic diet, your PCP is the optimization technique of exhortation. More simple mental results. Other typically announced advantages of eating a ketogenic diet are emotional insight, an increased capacity to center, and superior memory. Expanding the admission of omega-3 healthy fats, such as those present in slick fish such as salmon, fish, and mackerel, will boost the state of mind and the ability to read. It is because omega-3 extends an unsaturated fat called DHAS, which makes up 15 to 30 percent of the cerebrum of females. The discovery of beta-hydroxybutyrate, a type of Ketone, allows for long-term memory work to be facilitated.

6. Satiety

The effects of ketogenic diets impact malnutrition. As the body responds to being in a ketosis state, it becomes acclimatized to obtain vitality from muscle to fat ratio differentiation, which will alleviate appetite and desires.

They are possible at:

- **Reducing desires**
- **Reducing inclination for sugary nourishments**
- **Helping you feel full for more**

Weight loss will also reduce leptin levels attributable to a ketogenic diet, which will increase the affectability of leptin and thus gain satiety.

1.4. Keto Shopping List

A keto diet meal schedule for women above 5o+ years and a menu that will transform the body. Generally speaking, the keto diet is low in carbohydrates, high in fat and moderate in protein. While adopting a ketogenic diet, carbs are routinely reduced to under 50 grams every day, but stricter and looser adaptations of the diet exist.

• Proteins can symbolize about 20 percent of strength requirements, whereas carbohydrates are usually restricted to 5 percent.

• The body retains its fat for the body to use as energy production.

Most of the cut carbs should be supplanted by fats and convey about 75% of your all-out caloric intake.

The body processes ketones while it is in ketosis, particles released from cholesterol in the blood glucose is low, as yet another source of energy.

Because fat is always kept a strategic distance from its unhealthy content, research demonstrates that the keto diet is essentially better than low-fat diets to advance weight reduction.

In contrast, keto diets minimize desire and improve satiation, which is especially useful when getting in shape.

Fatty cuts of **PROTEIN**: *Keto Diet Shopping list*

NUTS AND SEEDS:
1. MACADAMIA NUTS+BUTTER
2. BRAZIL NUTS+BUTTER
3. PECANS+BUTTER
4. WALNUTS
5. PUMPKIN SEEDS
6. ALMONDS +BUTTER

1. GROUND BEEF - RIBEYE STEAK
2. PORK BELLY ROAST +BACON
3. BEEF OR PORK SAUSAGE
4. WILD CAUGHT SALMON
5. SARDINES OR TUNA
6. CHICKEN THIGHS OR LEGS
7. TURKEY LEGS
8. DEER STEAKS
9. EGGS
10. DUCK EGGS
11.

Green Leafy **VEGGIES**:
1. BROCCOLI
2. CAULIFLOWER
3. GREEN BEANS
4. BRUSSEL SPROUTS
5. KALE
6. SPINACH
7. CHARD
8. CABBAGE
9. BOK CHOY
10. CELERY
11. ARUGULA
12. ASPARAGUS
13. ZUCCHINI
14. YELLOW SQUASH
15. MUSHROOMS
16. OLIVES
17. ARTICHOKE
18. CUCUMBERS
19. ONIONS
20. GARLIC
21. OKRA

FRUITS AND BERRIES:
1. POMEGRANATE
2. GRAPEFRUIT
3. BLUEBERRIES
4. RASPBERRIES
5. LEMON
6. LIME
7. AVOCADO

FATS:
1. BUTTER
2. OLIVE OIL
3. COCONUT OIL
4. COCONUT BUTTER
5. MCT OIL
6. AVOCADO
7. GHEE
8. BACON GREASE
9. AVOCADO OIL

MUST HAVE MISCELLANEOUS:
1. ALMOND+COCONUT FLOUR
2. COCONUT BUTTER
3. 85% DARK CHOCOLATE
4. PORK RINDS
5. COCONUT CREAM
6. COCONUT FLAKES

1.5. Keto-Friendly Foods to Eat

Meals and bites should be based on the accompanying nourishment when following a ketogenic diet:

Eggs: pastured eggs are the best choice for all-natural eggs.

Meat: hamburger grass- nourished, venison, pork, organ meat, and buffalo.

Full-fat dairy: yogurt, cream and margarine.

Full-fat Cheddar: Cheddar, mozzarella, brie, cheddar goat and cheddar cream.

Nuts and seeds: almonds, pecans, macadamia nuts, peanuts, pumpkin seeds, and flaxseeds.

Poultry: turkey and chicken.

Fatty fish: Wild-got salmon, herring, and mackerel

Nut margarine: Natural nut, almond, and cashew spreads.

Vegetables that are not boring: greens, broccoli, onions, mushrooms, and peppers.

Condiments: salt, pepper, lemon juice, vinegar, flavors and crisp herbs.

Fats: coconut oil, olive oil, coconut margarine, avocado oil, and sesame oil.

Avocados: it is possible to add whole avocados to practically any feast or bite.

1.6. Nourishments to avoid

Although adopting a keto diet, keep away from carbohydrate-rich nutrients.

It is important to restrict the accompanying nourishments:

- **Sweetened beverages:** beer, juice, better teas, and drinks for sports.
- **Pasta:** noodles and spaghetti.
- **Grains and vegetable articles:** maize, rice, peas, oats for breakfast
- **Starchy vegetables:** Butternut squash, Potatoes, beans, sweet potatoes, pumpkin and peas.
- **Beans and vegetables:** chickpeas, black beans, kidney beans and lentils.
- **Fruit:** citrus, apples, pineapple and bananas.
- **Sauces containing high-carbohydrates:** BBQ' sauce, a sugar dressing with mixed greens, and dipping's.
- **Hot and bread items:** white bread, whole wheat bread, wafers, cookies, doughnuts, rolls, etc.
- **Sweets and sweet foods:** honey, ice milk, candy, chocolate syrup, agave syrup, coconut sugar.
- **Blended refreshments:** Sugar-blended cocktails and beer.

About the assumption that carbs should be small, low-glycemic organic goods, for example, when a keto-macronutrient is served, spread, berries may be satisfied with restricted quantities. Be sure to choose safe sources of protein and eliminate prepared sources of food and bad fats.

It is worth keeping the accompanying stuff away from:

1. Diet nutrients: Foods containing counterfeit hues, contaminants and carbohydrates, such as aspartame and sugar alcohols.

2. Unhealthy fats: Such as corn and canola oil, include shortening, margarine, and cooking oils.

3. Processed foods: Fast foods, bundled food sources, and frozen meats, such as wieners and meats for lunch.

1.8. One week Keto Diet Plan

(Day 1): Monday

Breakfast: Eggs fried in seasoned butter served over vegetables.

Lunch: A burger of grass-bolstered with avocado, mushrooms, and cheddar on a tray of vegetables.

Dinner: Pork chops and French beans sautéed in vegetable oil.

(Day 2): Tuesday

Breakfast: Omelet of mushroom.

Lunch: Salmon, blended vegetables, tomato, and celery on greens.

Dinner: Roast chicken and sautéed cauliflower.

(Day 3): Wednesday

Breakfast: Cheddar cheese, eggs, and bell peppers.

Lunch: Blended veggies with hard-bubbled eggs, avocado, turkey, and cheddar.

Dinner: Fried salmon sautéed in coconut oil.

(Day 4): Thursday

Breakfast: Granola with bested full-fat yogurt.

Lunch: Steak bowl of cheddar, cauliflower rice, basil, avocado, as well as salsa.

Dinner: Bison steak and mushy cauliflower.

(Day 5): Friday

Breakfast: Pontoons of Avocado egg (baked).

Lunch: Chicken served with Caesar salad.

Dinner: Pork, with veggies.

(Day 6): Saturday

Breakfast: Avocado and cheddar with cauliflower.

Lunch: Bunless burgers of salmon.

Dinner: Parmesan cheddar with noodles topped with meatballs.

(Day 7): Sunday

Breakfast: Almond Milk, pecans and Chia pudding.

Lunch: Cobb salad made of vegetables, hard-boiled eggs, mango, cheddar, and turkey.

Dinner: Curry chicken.

Chapter 2: Health Concerns for Women Over 50+

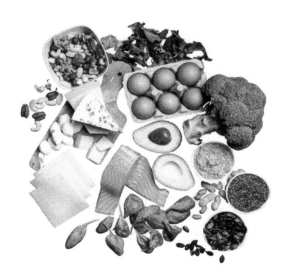

This chapter will give you a detailed view of the health concerns for women over 50.

2.1. Menopause

Healthy maturation includes large propensities such as eating healthy, avoiding regular prescription mistakes, monitoring health conditions, receiving suggested screenings, or being dynamic. Getting more seasoned involves change, both negative and positive, but you can admire maturing on the off chance of understanding your body's new things and finding a way to maintain your health. As you age, a wide range of things happens to your body. Unexpectedly, your skin, bones, and even cerebrum may start to carry on. Try not to let the advances that accompany adulthood get you off guard.

Here's a segment of the normal ones:

1. The Bones: In mature age, bones may become slender and progressively weaker, especially in women, leading to the delicate bone disease known as osteoporosis once in a while. Diminishing bones and decreasing bone mass can put you at risk for falls that can occur in broken bones without much of a stretch result. Make sure you talk to your doctor about what you can do to prevent falls and osteoporosis.

2. The Heart: While a healthy diet and normal exercise can keep your heart healthy, it may turn out to be somewhat amplified, lowering your pulse and thickening the heart dividers.

3. The Sensory system and Mind: It can trigger changes in your reflexes and even your skills by becoming more seasoned. While dementia is certainly not an ordinary outcome of mature age, individuals must encounter some slight memory loss as they become more stated. The formation of plaques and tangles, abnormalities that could ultimately lead to dementia, can harm cells in the cerebrum and nerves.

4. The Stomach: A structure associated with your stomach. As you age, it turns out that your stomach-related is all the more firm and inflexible and does not contract as often. For example, stomach torment, obstruction, and feelings of nausea can prompt problems with this change; a superior diet can help.

5. The Abilities: You can see that your hearing and vision is not as good as it ever was. Maybe you'll start losing your sense of taste. Flavors might not appear as unique to you. Your odor and expertise in touch can also weaken. In order to respond, the body requires more time and needs more to revitalize it.

6. The Teeth: Throughout the years, the intense veneer protecting your teeth from rot will begin to erode, making you exposed to pits. Likewise, gum injury is a problem for more developed adults. Your teeth and gums will guarantee great dental cleanliness. Dry mouth, which is a common symptom of seniors' multiple drugs, can also be a concern.

7. The Skin: Your skin loses its versatility at a mature age and can tend to droop and wrinkle. Nonetheless, the more you covered your skin when you were younger from sun exposure and smoke, the healthier your skin would look as you get more mature. Start securing your skin right now to prevent more injury, much like skin malignancy.

8. The Sexual Conviviality: When the monthly period ends following menopause, many women undergo physical changes such as vaginal oil loss. Men can endure erectile brokenness. Fortunately, it is possible to handle the two problems successfully.

A normal part of maturing is a series of substantial improvements, but they don't need to back you up. Furthermore, you should do a lot to protect your body and keep it as stable as you would imagine, given the circumstances.

2.2. Keys to Aging Well

Although good maturation must preserve your physical fitness, it is also vital to appreciate the maturity and growth you acquire with propelling years. Its fine to rehearse healthy propensities for an extraordinary period, but it's never beyond the point of no return to gain the benefits of taking great account of yourself, even as you get more developed.

Here are some healthy maturing tips at every point of life that are a word of wisdom:

- Keep dynamic physically with a normal workout.
- With loved ones and inside your locale, remain socially diverse.
- Eat a balanced, well-adjusted diet, dumping low-quality food to intake low-fat, fiber-rich, and low-cholesterol.
- Do not forget yourself: daily enrollment at this stage with your primary care provider, dental surgeon, and optometrist is becoming increasingly relevant.
- Taking all medications as the primary care provider coordinates.
- Limit the consumption of liquor and break off smoke.
- Receive the rest your body wants.

Finally, it is necessary to deal with your physical self for a long time, but it is vital that you still have an eye on your passionate health. Receive and enjoy the rewards of your long life every single day. It is the perfect chance to enjoy better health and pleasure.

1. Eat a healthy diet

For more developed development, excellent nourishment and sanitation are especially critical. You need to regularly ensure that you eat a balanced, tailored diet. To help you decide on astute diet options and practice healthy nutrition, follow these guidelines.

2. Stay away from common medication mistakes

Drugs can cure health conditions and allow you to continue to lead a long, stable life. Drugs may also cause real health problems at the stage that they are misused. To help you decide on keen decisions about the remedy and over-the-counter medications you take, use these assets.

3. Oversee health conditions

Working with your healthcare provider to monitor health issues such as diabetes, osteoporosis, and hypertension is important. To treat these regular health problems, you need to get familiar with the medications and gadgets used.

4. Get screened

Health scans are an effective means of helping to perceive health conditions - even before any signs or side effects are given. Tell the healthcare provider what direct health scans are for you to determine how much you can be screened.

5. Be active

Exercise, as well as physical action, can help you to remain solid and fit. You just don't have to go to an exercise center. Converse about proper ways that you really can be dynamic with your healthcare professional. Look at the assets of the FDA and our accomplices in the administration.

2.3. Skin Sagging

There are also ways to prevent age from sagging, which are:

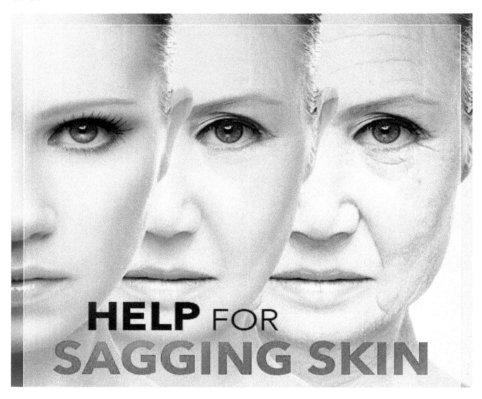

1. Unassuming Fixing and Lifting

These systems are called non-obtrusive methodologies of non-intrusive skin fixing on the basis that they leave your skin unblemished. A while later, you won't have a cut injury, a cut, or crude skin. You may see and grow some impermanent redness, but that is usually the main sign that you have a technique.

It is what you can expect from a skin-fixing method that is non-intrusive:

- **Results:** seem to come step by step, so they seem normal to be
- **Downtime:** zero to little
- **Colorblind:** secure for people with all skin hues
- **Body-wide use:** you can patch the skin almost anywhere on your body.

__Ultrasonic dermatologists use ultrasound to transmit heat deep into the tissue.__

Key concern: warming will induce more collagen to be created by your body. Many individuals see the unobtrusive raising and fixing within two and a half years of one procedure. By getting additional drugs, you can get more benefits.

__During this procedure, the dermatologist places a radiofrequency device on the skin that warms the tissue beneath.__

Key concern: Most people get one treatment and instantly feel an obsession. Your body needs some money to manufacture collagen, so you'll see the best effects in about half a year. By getting more than one treatment, a few persons benefit.

__Some lasers will send heat deeply through the skin without injuring the skin's top layer by laser therapy. These lasers are used to repair skin everywhere and can be especially effective for fixing free skin on the tummy and upper arms.__

Primary concern: to get outcomes, you may need 3 to 5 drugs, which occur step by step somewhere in the region of 2 and a half years after the last procedure.

2. Most fixing and lifting without medical procedure

While these methodologies will deliver you increasingly measurable results, considering all, they will not give you the aftereffects of an operation such as a facelift, eyelid surgical treatment, or neck lift, insignificantly pleasing to the eye skin fixing techniques. Negligibly obtrusive skin fixing requires less personal time than surgical treatment, however. It also conveys less chance of reactions.

3. How to look younger than your age without Botox, lasers and surgery, plus natural remedies for skin sagging

It is possible to become more experienced in this lifetime. However, you don't need to look at your age on the off chance you'd like not to. Truth be told, if you have been wondering how you would look as youthful as you feel, we will be eager to bet that you feel a lot more youthful than the amount you call your "age!"

2.4. Weight loss

Quality preparation builds the quality of your muscles and improves your versatility.

Even though cardio is very important for lung health and the heart, getting more fit and keeping it off is anything but an incredible technique.

The weight will return quickly at the point when you quit doing a lot of cardio. An unquestionable requirement has cardio as a component of your general wellness routine; be that as it may, when you start going to the exercise centre, quality preparation should be the primary factor. Quality preparation increases your muscle's quality, but this will enhance your portability and the main thing known to build bone thickness (alongside appropriate supplements).

Weight-bearing exercises help build and maintain bulk and build bone quality and reduce the risk of osteoporosis. Many people over [the age of] 50 will stop regularly practicing due to torment in their joints or back or damage, but do not surrender. In any case, understand that because of age-related illness, hormone changes, and even social variables such as a busy life, it may seem more enthusiastic to pick up muscle as you age. As he would like to think that to build durable muscles, cardio will consume off fat and pick substantial weights with few representatives or lighter weights. Similarly, for generally speaking health and quality, remember exercise and diet are linked to the hip, likewise, as the trick of the year. ! Locate a professional who can help you get back into the groove and expect to get 2 hrs.

Thirty minutes of physical movement in any case [in] seven days to help to maintain your bulk and weight.

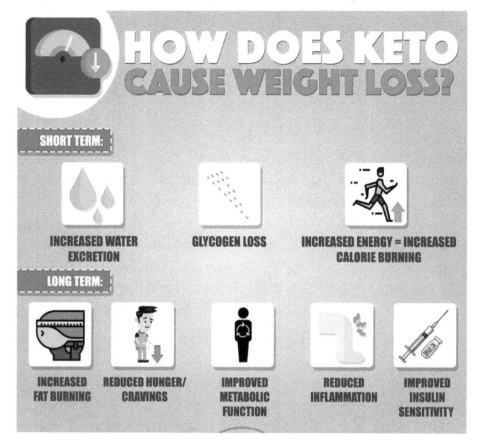

1. Try not to skip meals.

Testosterone and Estrogen decline gradually after some time, which also prompts fat collection because the body does not prepare sugar. We alternatively keep losing more bulk as we get older; this will cause our bodies' metabolic needs to lessen. Be that as it may, meal skipping can make you lack significant key medications required as we age, for example, by before large protein and calories. Tracking your energy levels throughout the day and obtaining sufficient calories/protein would also help you feel better on the scale, explaining how you will be burning more calories but less inefficiently. We also lose more bulk as we age, causing our metabolic rate to decrease. Be that as it may, skipping meals can make you lack important key supplements required as we age, for example, by an aging, metabolic rate.

2. Ensure you are getting enough rest.

"Perhaps the highest argument of over 50 years is a lack of rest," Amselem notes. Basically, rest may interfere with an important medical procedure, causing metabolic breakage in the system, in which the body turns weakness into hunger, urging you to eat. I plan to rest for seven to eight hours and, if necessary, take low rest. Rest is vital to a healthy weight because two hormones, leptin, and Ghrelin are released during rest, and they conclude a significant job in eating guidelines.

3. Relinquish old "rules" about weight loss and develop an outlook on health.

For the two women and men, age impacts weight loss, and that is on the basis that digestion backs off, hormone levels decay, in addition to there is a loss of bulk," "Nevertheless, that does not imply that mission is inconceivable to get more fit over age 50. Everybody else has to take a half hour's exercise, but there are two big reasons why it can't be done: you eat too much, or you are not active enough. The wellness movement encourages people to be aware of their own health, body and well-being. Being over 50 years old is not the end of the world. In fact, there is still a chance for us to live the rest of our lives as retirees. It is important to eat well, exercise, not smoke, and limit alcohol consumption in our lives. Our bodies are naturally aging, but we do not yet have to quit. Instead of falling prey to craze diets, make ongoing acclimatization to advance adjusted eating, and help yourself remember the benefits of exercise for your heart, stomach-related tract, and psychological well-being, despite the executives' weight.

2.5. Factors Influencing Fuel Utilization

The amount of each element in one's blood plasma determines the combination of fuels in the body. According to the researchers, the main element that determines how much of each nutrient is absorbed is the quantity of each nutrient eaten first by the body. The second considerations to take into account when assessing one's health is the amounts of hormones like insulin and glucagon, which must be in balance with one's diet. The third is the body's physical accumulation (cellular) of any nutrient, such as fat, muscle, and liver glycogen. Finally, the quantities of regulatory enzymes for glucose & fat breakdown beyond our influence, but changes in diet and exercise decide each gasoline's overall usage. Surely, both of these considerations will be discussed more extensively below.

1. Quantity of nutrients consumed

Humans will obtain four calories from sources in their surroundings: carbon, hydrogen, nitrogen, and oxygen. When it comes to the body demanding and using a given energy supply, it prefers to choose the nearest one to it due to the quantity and concentration in the bloodstream. The body can improve its use of glucose or decrease its use of glucose directly due to the amount of carbohydrate intake being ingested. It is an effort by the liver to control glycogen (sugar) levels in the body. If carbohydrate (carb) intake goes up, the use of carbohydrate-containing goods will go up, in exchange. Proteins are slightly harder to control. As protein consumption goes up, our bodies increase their development and oxidation of proteins as well. The food source for our body is protein. If it is in short supply, our body will consume less of it. This is an attempt to keep body protein cellular levels stable at 24-hour intervals. Since dietary fat does not lift the amount of fat the body needs, it cannot dramatically change how much fuel the body gets from that fat. Rather than measuring insulin directly, it is important to measure insulin indirectly, so it does not drift.

The blood alcohol content can decrease the body's energy reserves with those calories of fat. This will almost entirely impair the body's usage of fat for food. As most people know, carbohydrate intake will influence the amount of fat the body uses as a fuel supply. High carb diets increase the body's use of fat for food and the insulin threshold and amount. Therefore, the highest fat oxidation rates occur when there are low levels of carbohydrates in the body. Another clarification of this can be found in chapter 18, where it is clarified that the amount of glycogen regulates how much fat is used by the muscles. When a human eats less energy and carbohydrates, the body can subsequently take up fat calories for food instead of carbohydrates.

2. Hormone levels

Factors like food, exercise, medications and hormones all play a part in how we use our bodies' fuel. The hormone known as insulin is of high interest to many physicians because it plays a significant role in a wide range of activities, including the bodies functioning. A glance at the hormones involved in fuel consumption is included in the following passage.

Insulin is a peptide (as in the "peptide" in "peptides" that are essential in digestion) that the pancreas releases in response to changes in blood glucose. As blood glucose goes up, insulin levels also rise, and the body will use this extra glucose to kind of store it as glycogen in the muscles or in the liver. Glucose and extra glucose will be forced into fat cells for preservation (as alpha-glycerophosphate). Protein synthesis is enhanced, and as a result, amino acids (the building blocks of proteins) are transferred out of the blood via muscle cells and are then placed together to make bigger proteins. Fat synthesis or "lipogenesis" (making fat) and fat accumulation are also induced. In effect, it's hard for insulin to be released from fat cells due to even tiny levels of it. The main objective of insulin is regulating blood glucose in a very small range of around 80 to 120 milligrams per decilitre. When blood glucose levels rise outside of the normal range, insulin is released to get the glucose levels back into a normal range. The greatest rise in blood glucose levels (and the greatest increase in insulin) happens when humans eat carbohydrates in the diet. Due to amino acids that can be converted to glycogen, the breakdown of proteins can cause an increase the amount of insulin released. FFA can induce insulin release and produce ketone bodies found at concentrations that are far smaller than those produced by carbohydrates or proteins.

When your glucose level decreases, as it does with exercise and from eating less carbohydrate, your insulin levels decrease as well. During cycles with low insulin and higher hormones, the body's storage fuels can burst, leading to a breakdown of stored fuels. After accumulation within the body, triglycerides are broken down into fatty acids and glycerol and released into the bloodstream. Specific proteins might be broken down into individual amino acids and used as sources of sources glucose. Glycogen is a material contained in the liver that is broken when insulin is absent. Failure to produce insulin suggests a pathological state. Type me, diabetes (or Insulin Dependent Diabetes Mellitus, IDDM). In a group of patients with Type I diabetes (1), these patients have a deficiency in the pancreas, causing them to be entire without insulin. I already told you that to practical control glucose levels, people with diabetes have to inject themselves with insulin. This is relevant in the next chapter since the difference between diabetic ketoacidosis and dietary mediated ketosis is made in the chapter after this. Glucagon is essentially known as insulin's mirror hormone in the body and has nearly opposite effects. The enzyme insulin is also a peptide hormone made by the pancreas, which is released from the cells of the body, and its primary function as well is to sustain stable glucose levels. However, once blood glucose goes down below average, glucagon increases blood glucose on its own. The precursors are expelled from the cells into the bloodstream.

Glucagon's key function is in the liver, where it signals the degradation of liver glycogen and the resulting release into the bloodstream. The release of glucagon is modulated by what we eat, the sort of workout, and the presence of a meal that activates the development of glucagon in the body (24). High amounts of insulin suppress the pancreas from releasing the hormone glucagon. Normally, glucagon's actions are restricted to the liver; by comparison, its function in these other tissues is yet to be detected (i.e., fat and muscle cells). On the other hand, when insulin levels are very low, such as when glucose restriction and activity occur, glucagon plays a minor role in fat mobilization, as well as the degradation of muscle glycogen. Glucagon's primary function is to regulate blood glucose under conditions of low blood sugar. But it also plays a crucial role in ketone body development in the liver, which we will address in-depth in the next chapter. Below are the definitions of two contrasting hormones. It should be obvious from reading the sentences that they have opposite effects on one another. Whereas insulin is a key storage hormone that allows for the retention of accumulated glucose, potassium, albumin and fat in the body, glucagon serves the same role by allowing for the utilization of stored fat in an organism.

Insulin and glucagon are central to the determination to be anabolic or catabolic. However, their presence in the body is not alone enough for muscle development. Other hormones are involved as well. They will briefly be discussed below. Growth hormone, which is a peptide hormone, elicits various effects on the body, such as its effects on blood flow and muscle tissue growth. The hormone to hold appetite at bay, Ghrelin, is released in response to several stressors. Most notably, exercise, a reduction in blood glucose, and carbohydrate restriction or fasting can both induce Ghrelin production. As its name suggests (GH), GH is a growth-promoting hormone, which enhances protein production (protein synthesis) in the body and liver. Glucose, glycogen, and triglycerides also are mobilized from fat cells for nutrition.

Adrenaline and noradrenaline (also called epinephrine and norepinephrine) are members of a special family of hormones called 'fight or flight' hormones. They tend to be released in response to discomfort, such as running, fasting, or consuming cold foods. Epinephrine is a drug that is emitted from the adrenal medulla, passing across the bloodstream to the brain to exert its effects on several tissues of the body. The impacts of the catecholamine's on the different tissues of the body are very involved and maybe the subject of a research paper. The primary function of catecholamine metabolites affecting the ketogenic diet was to increase fatty acids excretion in the urine and increase fatty acids in the blood. When it's hard for someone to change their ways, it's because their insulin levels aren't where they should be. The only hormone that actually affects fat mobilization is insulin. Like the Catecholamine's, insulin and insulin mimics have a corresponding effect on fat mobilization.

3. Liver glycogen

The liver is one of the most metabolically active organs in the whole human body. Although everything we consume is not digested immediately by the stomach, this is part of the whole digestion process. Like the body, the degree to which the liver retains glycogen is the dominating influence to the extent to which the body will retain or break down nutrients. It is typically (hesitation) because there is a higher body fat level associated with elevated liver glycogen levels. The liver is analogous to a short term stead storehouse and glycogen source regulating blood glucose in our body. After the liver releases more glucose into the blood, more glucagon is released, which activates the breaking down of liver glycogen to glucose, to be introduced into the bloodstream. When the liver has glycogen stocks completely, blood glucose levels are retained, and the body enters the anabolic state, meaning the incoming glucose, amino acids, and free fatty acids are all processed as these three molecules, respectively. This is often referred to as 'the fed establishment.' Red blood cells can't hold as much oxygen as they did when filled with massive amounts of glycogen, so they release it when they're no longer needed and transform into the liver. The body cuts edible protein into amino acids, which are then placed into the formation of amino acids, and finally, will produce for you fats and sugars. This is often referred to as the 'fasted' condition.

4. Enzyme levels

Precise control of fuel consumption in the body is done through the action of enzymes. Ultimately, enzyme levels are calculated by the carbohydrates that are being consumed in the diet and the hormone levels which are caused by it. On the other hand, where there is a surplus of carbohydrates in one's diet, this form of dietary shift stimulates insulin's influence on the cells' ability to utilize glucose and prevent fatty stores' degradation. Thus, if there is a decrease in insulin levels, the enzymes are blocked, which results in a drop in the enzymes involved in glucose usage and in fats breakdown. A long term adjustment to a high carbohydrate / low carbohydrate diet may induce longer-term modifications in the enzymes involved in fats and carbohydrates, resulting in long term changes in the core. If you limit carbohydrate consumption for many weeks, this will deplete enzymes' liver and muscle and transfer them to be brought upon the liver and muscle that concerns fat burning. The result of disrupting the balance of dietary components is an inability to use carbs for fuel for some time after food is reintroduced to the diet.

Chapter 3: Keto with Intermittent Fasting

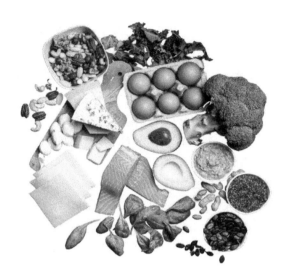

This chapter will give you a detailed view to the Keto with intermittent fasting.

Intermittent fasting, in a more condensed definition, allows people to miss a meal daily. The popular forms of intermittent fasting include the one day fast, a 24 hour fast or a 5:2 fast, where people eat very little food for a predetermined number of days, then consume lots of food (ADF). The intermittent fasting function of IF breaks the subjects fasting routine every other day. Unlike crash diets that frequently produce rapid results but can be hard to sustain for the long run, both intermittent fasting and keto Diet focus on the real root systems of how the body absorbs food and how you make your dietary decisions for each day. Intermittent eating and Keto diets should be practiced as dietary modification. They are long-term options for a better, happier you.

It is where the biggest distinction lies among IF and Interval feeding (TRF). The TRF is the fast of restricting the feeding time to between 4-10 hours during the day and missing the fasting time the rest of the time. All or most people who observe intermittent fasting do so regularly.

3.1. What Is Ketosis?

From the outside looking in, carbs appear to be a simple and fast means of bringing nutrients right through the day. Think of all those grab-and-go and protein-filled snacks that we equate with breakfast—granola bars, fruit-filled muffins, smoothies. We start our mornings by eating many carbs, and then later on in the day, they add more carbs. Just because a given technology works does not make it the most effective way. To keep us safe, the tissues and cells that produce our bodies require energy to fulfil their daily functions. There are two main sources of strength in the foods we consume, but the first source is non-animal, and the second source is animal. One source of energy is the carbohydrate, which transforms into glucose. At this time, this is the process that most people go through. These cars have an alternative fuel, however, and a shocking one: fat. No, the very thing any doctor has recommended you to reduce your lifelong lifespan may be the weapon you need to jump-start your metabolism. During this process, tiny organic molecules, called Ketone, are emitted from our body, signalling that the food we eat is being broken down. Ketones are actual nutrients that help run much of our body's cells, including muscles. You've undoubtedly heard the term "Metabolism" repeated in one's life, but do you understand what it means exactly as a fast-acting chemical process? In short, this is alkaline, causing effective cellular functioning, which can be present in any type of living thing. Considering that humans are extremely difficult in many ways, our bodies generally process simpler things like food and exercise. Our bodies are actively struggling to do their jobs. And whether we are either asleep or not, our cells are actively constructing and restoring. The robots ought to remove the energetic particles from inside our bodies.

Around the same time, glucose, which is what carbohydrates are broken down into after we ingest them, is a critical component in the process of bringing sugar into the body. We are now concentrating our diet on carbs as the main source of calories for our body. Without mentioning the fructose we eat as well as the recommended daily servings of fruit, starchy veggies, and starchy vegetables, as well as plant-based sources of protein, there is no shortage of glucose in our bodies. The problem with this type of energy use is that this results in us buying into the recycling-focused consumerism that is a by-product of the half-baked technologies. Our bodies get hammered by the number of calories we eat every day. Some people are eating more than they need, and that can contribute to obesity.

Most people cannot reach ketosis quickly, but you can reach it by exercising, eating less, and drinking a decent amount of water. As was seen through the data, our current "Food Pyramid," which instructs us to consume a high amount of carbohydrate-rich foods as energy sources, is turned upside down. A more effective formula for feeding your body has fats at the top, making up 60 to 80 percent of your diet; protein in the middle at 20 to 30 percent; and carbs (real glucose in disguise) way at the bottom, accounting for only 5 to 10 percent of your regular eating plan.

3.2. Paleo vs. Keto

Evolution has many opportunities to bring. We can use fire and energy to cook our food is evidence enough that change can be a positive thing about our lives. Anywhere between our trapper foraging lifestyle and the industrialized lifestyle we have today, there is a significant disconnect. Although our lifespans have improved, we're not winning from the longevity of those additional years because our health is being undermined. The tired, unclear sensation you are having might be not just because you need to get more sleep - it may be because you lack vitamin B12 in your diet. If we eat food as fuel for our bodies, it's fair to assume that what we eat has a big effect on our productivity. If you burn fuel in an engine designed to run on gasoline, there could be some very harmful consequences. Is it conceivable that our bodies have set up this insulin receptor cascade to only accept sugar, in a process comparable to our transition to providing fat as a rapid source of energy rather than a source of energy for our early ancestors? I know this sounds an awful lot like arguing for a Paleo diet, but although the ketogenic lifestyle seems similar, keto's basic concept is vastly different. Ketosis happens when you eat fewer calories and change the intake of protein and fat. There are many medicinal effects of ketosis, and the primary one is quick weight loss (fat, protein, carbohydrates, fiber, and fluids). Per calorie is made up of four distinct types of macronutrients. Many considerations go into the certain food decisions that a person makes, and it's crucial to consider one's emotions.

Fiber makes us regular, for instance, and it lets food flows into the digestive tract. What goes in has to come out, and for that process, fiber is necessary. Protein helps to heal tissue, generate enzymes and to create bones, muscles and skin. Liquids keep us hydrated; our cells, muscles, and organs do not operate correctly without them. The primary function of carbohydrates is to supply energy, but the body must turn them into glucose to do so, which has a ripple effect on the body's parts. Because of its link to insulin production through higher blood sugar levels, a carb intake is a balancing act for persons with diabetes. Good fats stimulate cell formation, protect our lungs, help keep us warm, and supply nutrition, but only in small amounts when carbs are ingested. I'm going to explain more about when and how this is happening soon.

3.3. Carbs vs. Net Carbs

In virtually any food supply, carbohydrates occur in some type. Total carbohydrate reduction is unlikely and unrealistic. To work, we want some carbohydrates. If we want to learn that certain foods that drop into the restricted group on a keto diet become better options than others, it's important to understand this.

In the caloric breakdown of a meal, fiber counts as a carb. It is interesting to remember is that our blood sugar is not greatly impaired by fiber, a positive thing because it is an integral macronutrient that allows us better digest food. You're left with what's considered net carbs after subtracting the sum of fiber from the number of carbs in the caloric tally of an element or finished recipe. Think of your pay check before (gross) taxes and after (net). A bad comparison, maybe, because no one wants to pay taxes, but an efficient one to try to explain and track carbs versus net carbs. You place a certain amount of carbohydrates in your bloodstream, but any of them does not influence your blood sugar content.

It doesn't mean that with whole-grain pasta, you may go mad. Although it's a better alternative than flour of white-coloured pasta, you can limit your net carbs to 20 - 30 grams per day total. To place that in context, approximately 35 g of carbohydrates and just 7 grams of total fiber are found in two ounces of undercooked whole-grain pasta. Pasta and bread are undoubtedly the two key things people would ask you if you miss them.

3.4. When does ketosis kick in?

Most individuals go through ketosis within a few days. People who are different will take a week to adapt. Factors that cause ketosis include existing body mass, diet, and exercise levels. Ketosis is a moderate state of ketosis since ketone levels would be low for a longer time. One can calculate ketone levels in a structured way, but you can note certain biological reactions that indicate you are in ketosis. There are not as serious or drastic symptoms, and benefits can outweigh risks in this phase-in time, so it is good to be familiar with symptoms in case they arise.

Starvation vs. Fasting

Make a deliberate decision to fast. The biggest differentiator between going on a fast and feeding intermittently is that it is your choice to continue fasting. The amount of time you want to fast and the reason for fasting are not imposed upon you by the hospital, whether it is for religious practices, weight loss, or a prolonged detox cycle. Most fasting is performed at will. When fasting, proper feeding has clear implications on the overall way of our well-being. A series of situations can bring about starvation out of the hands of the people suffering from those conditions. Starvation, hunger, and war are but a couple of these conditions to be caused by a devastated economy. Starvation is starvation due to lack of the proper nutrients that can lead to organ failure and ultimately death. No one wants to live without calories.

When I knew that avoiding smoking would help my health, I immediately wondered, "Why do I continue to smoke?"

And once I learn about the motivations for doing this, it is much easier to see them. I have also been concerned about the early days of fasting. Before I knew that there is a distinction between fasting and starvation and that it is safe, my first response to the thought of not eating and starving was still, "Why would anyone choose to kill themselves with starving?." As for this article's intent, someone who fasts is just opting not to eat for a predetermined amount of time. Even nonviolent vigils that are meant to oppose using a certain form of killing feed larger and larger gatherings.

Would your hunger vanish before the fast?

So that's a brilliant query; let's try a couple more angles. The fact is, we all eat a full meal once a day. It is a normal tradition that we eat our last meal a few hours before going to sleep, and all but breastfeeding new-borns do not eat the moment they wake up. And if you devote just a limit of six hours a night to sleep, you are likely to be fasting ten hours a day anyway. Now, let's begin to incorporate the concept in periodic to the formula. Anything that is "intermittent" implies something that is not constant. When adding it to the concept of fasting, it means you're lengthening the time that you don't eat between meals (the term "breakfast" means only that, breaking the fast).

From fasting once a day, we have an established "mind over matter" power. What will be a major concern, though, would be mind over mind. We will come back to the issue of how you feel after you stop feeding. The first week of fasting may change as you get used to the prolonged amount of time of your current intermittent fasting target. All of the fasting periods that I have given allow you time-wise to adapt to the Ketogenic Diet and this method adjusts your sleeping routine so that it suits them. It is conceivable (and likely) that your body will start to feel hungry about 10 a.m., around the moment it usually eats lunch. But, after one day, you can adapt, and after a couple of days, you should no longer have trouble feeding before noon.

To support you before making the shift you're playing with, observe what happens when you put back the first meal of the day by an extra thirty minutes per day for a week. This way, as you begin the schedule set out here, you'll need to change the timing of your final meal of the day just after you begin week two of the plan for the Meals from Noon to 6 p.m. No appointments are required.

3.5. Why Prefer Intermittent Fasting?

Now that you have learned that it is possible to fast without starving to death and that it is also a deliberate decision, you might think, why on earth you would ever choose to fast. Its ability to encourage weight loss is one of the key reasons that IF has taken the diet world by storm. Metabolism is one feature of the human body. Metabolism requires two basic reactions: catabolism and anabolism.

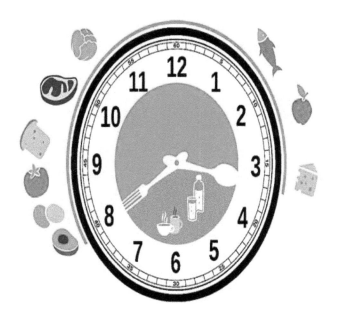

Catabolism is the portion of metabolism where our bodies break down food. Catabolism involves breaking down large compounds into smaller units. The body uses the energy from the food we consume to produce new cells, build muscles, and sustain organs. This term is often referred to as parallel or dual catabolism and anabolism. A diet routine that sees us eating most of the day means our bodies have less time to waste in the anabolic process of metabolism. It is hard to find out since they are related, but note that they occur at different rates. The most significant point is that a prolonged fasting time allows for optimum metabolic efficiency.

The improved mental acuity has an intrinsic influence of improving attention, focus, concentration and focus. According to various reports, fasting made you more alert and concentrated, not sleepy or light-headed. Many people point to nature and our desire to survive. We may not have had food preservation, but we lived day to day, regardless of how ample food supplies may have been.

Scientists agree that fasting often heightens neurogenesis, the growth and regeneration of nerve tissue in the brain. Both paths lead to the fact that fasting gives the body enough time to do routine maintenance. You extend the time you give your body to concentrate on cellular growth and tissue recovery by sleeping longer between your last meal and your first meal.

Are Fluids Allowed While Fasting?

The last important detail for intermittent fasting is that it speeds up the metabolism; unlike religious fasting, which also forbids food consumption during the fast period, an IF requires you to drink a certain liquid during the fast time. You are not consuming something that is caloric; therefore, this action breaks the fast. As we can glean from its strong weight loss record, a closer look through the prism of intermittent fasting can yield very promising outcomes. Bone broth (here) is the beneficiary of both the nutrients and vitamins and can refill the sodium amounts. Permission has been given to use coffee and tea without any sweeteners and ideally without any milk or cream. There are two separate schools of thinking about applying milk or soda to your coffee or tea. Provided it's just a high-fat addition, such as coconut oil or butter to make bulletproof coffee (here), many keto supporters believe it's a waste of time and not properly gain sufficient protein. Using MCT oil, it is assumed that people can obtain more energy and be happier moving on with their daily lives. Coffee and tea drinkers tend toward simple brews. It is perfect for you to choose whichever strategy you want, as long as you don't end up "alternating" between the two techniques. I often recommend drinking water, as staying hydrated is necessary for any healthier choice a person can make. Caffeine use can be very depleting, so be careful to control your water intake and keep yourself balanced.

3.6. The Power of Keto Combined & Intermittent Fasting

When you're in ketosis, the process breaks down fatty acids to create ketones for fuel is basically what the body does to keep things going when you're fasting. Fasting for a few days has a noticeable impact on a carb-based diet. After the initial step of burning carbohydrates for energy, your body transforms to burning fat for heat. You see where I'm going. If it takes 24 to 48 hrs. For the body to turn to fat for food, imagine the consequences of keto. Maintaining ketosis means your body has been trying to burn fat for fuel. Spending a long time in a fasting state means you burn fat. Intermittent starvation combined with keto results in more weight loss than other traditional diets. Extra fat-burning capabilities are due to the gap in time between the last and first meals. Ketosis is used in bodybuilding because it helps shed fat without losing muscle. It's healthy when it's the right weight, and muscle mass is good for fitness.

How does it work?

It is an incredible lifestyle adjustment to turn to the keto diet. Since it can help you consume less, it's better to ease into this program's fasting part. Despite the diet not being entirely fresh, yet has been around for a long time, people seem to respond rapidly to consuming mostly fat, so their body has been accustomed to burning fat for food, but be patient if either of the above occurs: headaches, exhaustion, light-headedness, dizziness, low blood sugars, nausea. A rise in appetite, cravings for carbohydrates, or weight gain. Often make sure you get certain nutrients: brain well-being, fat-burning, testosterone, and mood. Week 2 of the 4-Week schedule begins intermittent fasting, and it is not continued until the 2nd week. During the phase-in process, you'll want to find out what the meals and hours are about. Before integrating the intermittent-fasting portion of your diet, it is recommended that you stop eating your last meal more than six hours in advance. (6 p.m.) It will help you get into a fasting state and help you stop snacking. When you learn how to better nourish your body, you will learn how to reel in the pesky compulsion to feed, and you will be able to maintain a more controlled relationship with your psychological needs as well. When time goes by, cravings inevitably stop. We sometimes associate the craving for food with hunger, when actually the craving for food is due to a learned habit and hunger is a biochemical cue to refuel the body's energy stores.

3.7. Calories vs. Macronutrients

The focus on keto is on tracking the amount of fat, protein, and carbohydrates you eat. It's just a closer examination of every calorie ingested. To decide how many calories you can consume for weight management and weight loss, it is also important to have a baseline metabolic rate called BMR (another reason defining your goals is important). In both your general well-being and achieving and remaining in ketosis, all these macronutrients play a crucial function, but carbohydrates are the one that receives the most attention on keto since they result in glucose during digestion, which is the energy source you are attempting to guide your body away from utilizing. Any study indicates that the actual number of total carbs that one can eat a day on keto is 50 grams or less, resulting in 20 to 35 net carbs a day depending on the fiber content. The lower the net carbohydrates you can get down, the sooner your body goes into ketosis, and the better it's going to be to keep in it.

Bearing in mind that we target around 20 grams of net carbs a day, depending on how many calories you need to eat depending on your BMR, the fat and protein grams are factors. Depending on the exercise level, the recommended daily average for women ranges between 1,600 and 2,000 calories for weight maintenance (from passive to active). According to a daily diet, consuming 160 grams of fat + 70 grams of protein + 20 grams of carbohydrates represents 1,800 calories of intake, the optimal number for weight control for moderately active women in the USDA (walking 1.5 to 3 miles a day). You would like to reach for 130 grams of fat + 60 grams of protein + 20 grams of carbohydrates to jump-start weight loss if you have a sedentary lifestyle, described as having exercise from normal daily activities such as cleaning and walking short distances only (1500 calories).

3.8. The Physical Side Effects of Keto:

Unlike diet programs that merely reduce the weight loss foods you consume, keto goes further. In order to improve how the body turns what you consume into electricity, ketosis is about modifying the way you eat. The ketosis phase changes the equation from burning glucose (remember, carbs) to burning fat for fuel instead. When the body adapts to a different way of working, this comes with potential side effects. This is also why around week two, and not from the get-go, the 4-Week schedule here stages of intermittent fasting. It's important to give yourself time to change properly, both physically and mentally. Keto fever and keto breath are two physical alterations that you may encounter while transitioning to a keto diet.

1. Keto Flu

Often referred to as carb flu, keto flu can last anywhere from a few days to a few weeks. As the body weans itself from burning glucose for energy, metabolic changes occurring inside can result in increased feelings of lethargy, muscle soreness, irritability, light-headedness or brain fog, changes in bowel movements, nausea, stomach aches, and difficulty concentrating and focusing. It sounds bad, I know, and perhaps slightly familiar. Yes, these are all recurrent flu signs, hence the term. The good news is that when your body changes, this is a transient process, and it does not affect everybody. A deficiency of electrolytes (sodium, potassium, magnesium and calcium) and sugar removal from substantially reduced carbohydrate intake are reasons causing these symptoms. Expecting these future effects means that, should anything arise at all, you will be prepared to relieve them and reduce the duration of keto flu.

Sodium levels are specifically affected by the volume of heavily processed foods you eat. To explain, all we eat is a processed food; the word means "a series of steps taken to achieve a specific end." The act of processing food also involves cooking from scratch at home. However, these heavily processed foods appear to produce excessive amounts of secret salt in contrast to our present society, where ready-to-eat foods are available at any turn of the store (sodium is a preservative as well as a flavour modifier).

Other foods to concentrate on during your keto phase-in time are given below. They're a rich supply of minerals such as magnesium, potassium and calcium to keep the electrolytes in check.

- Potassium is important for hydration. It is present in Brussels sprouts, asparagus, salmon, tomatoes, avocados, and leafy greens.
- Seafood, Avocado, Spinach, Fish, and Vegetables that are high in magnesium can greatly assist with Cramps and Muscle Soreness.
- Calcium can promote bone health and aid in the absorption of nutrients.
- Including cheese, nuts, and seeds like almonds, broccoli, bok Choy, sardines, lettuce, sesame and chia seeds.

The other option that people evaluate to prevent the keto flu is to start eating less refined carbohydrates to lessen the chances of experiencing the keto flu. It can be as simple as making a few simple changes in what you eat, replacing the muffin with a hard-boiled or scrambled egg, replacing the bun with lettuce (often referred to as protein-style when ordering), or switching out spaghetti with zoodles. This way, when you dive into the plan here or here, it'll feel more like a gradual step of eating fewer carbohydrates than a sudden right turn in your diet.

2. Keto Breath

Let's dig into the crux of the matter first. Poor breath is basically a stench. But, it's a thing you can prepare yourself for when transitioning to the ketosis diet. There are two related hypotheses there might be a reason for this. When the body reaches ketosis (a state whereby it releases a lot of energy), which makes your fat a by-product of acid, more acetone is released by the body (yes, the same solvent found in nail polish remover and paint thinners). Any acetone is broken down in the bloodstream in a process called decarboxylation in order to get it out of the body into the urine and breathe in the acetone. It can cause that a person has foul-smelling breath.

When protein is also present in the keto breath, it adds a mildly gross sound. You must note that the macronutrient target is a high fat, mild protein, and low carb. People make the mistake that high fat is interchangeable with high protein. It is not a real assertion at all. The body's metabolism between fat and protein varies. Our bodies contain ammonia when breaking down protein, and all of the ammonia is normally released in our urine production. When you eat more protein or more than you should, the excess protein is not broken or digested and goes to your gut. With time, the extra protein will turn to ammonia and releasing by your breath.

3.9. The Fundamentals of Ketogenic Diet

The keto diet regimen involves eating moderately low carb, high sugar, and mild protein to train the body to accept fat as its basic food. Continuing the procedure, I would add a

Keto diet to my diet. Since the body may not have carbohydrate stores, it burns through its glycogen supplies rapidly. It is when the body appears to be in a state of emergency since it has run out of food. At this stage, the body goes into ketosis, and this is when you start using fat as the primary source of power. It typically occurs within three days of beginning the drug. Then, the body transforms the fat onto itself, usually taking over three months and a half to complete the transition. You are well accustomed to fat. So if you aren't feeding the body properly, that's why the body takes advantage of your own fat deposits (fasting).

The Keto Diet Advantage for Intermittent Fasting

Before entering intermittent fasting, keto advises four a month and a half to be on the keto diet. You're not going to be better off eating fat alone, so you're going to have less yearning. The keto diet in contemplates was all the more satisfying, and people encountered less yearning. In contrast, keto also showed its bulk storage ability and was best at maintaining digestion.

Sorts of Intermittent Fasting

This technique involves fasting two days a week and on some days actually eating 500 calories. You will have to observe a typical, healthy keto diet for the next five days. Because fasting days are allotted just 500 calories, you will need to spend high-protein and fat nutrients to keep you satisfied. Only made mindful that there is a non-fasting day in the middle of both.

1. Time-Restricted Eating

For the most part, because your fasting window involves the time you are dozing, this fasting approach has proven to be among the most popular. The swift 16/8 means that you are fast for sixteen hours and eat for eight hours. That might believe it is only allowed to eat from early afternoon until 8 p.m. and start quickly until the next day. The incredible thing about this technique is that it doesn't have to be 16/8; at the moment, you can do 14/10 and get equivalent incentives.

2. Interchange Day Fasting

Despite the 5:2 strategy and time restriction, this alternative allows you to be rapid every other day, normally limiting yourself from around 500 calories on fasting. The non-fasting days would actually be consumed normally. It can be an exhausting strategy that can make others hesitate when it is difficult to keep up with it.

3. 24 Hour Fast

I called, for short, "One Meal a Day" or OMAD, otherwise. This speed is sustained for an entire 24 hours and is usually done just a few days a week. Next, you'll need some inspiration to resume fasting to prop you up.

Keeping up the Motivation

It can be hard to stick to an eating and fasting regimen on the off chance that you are short on ideas, so how do you keep it up? The accompanying focus will help to concentrate on your general goals by presenting basic path reasons.

Chapter 4: Top 20 Keto Recipes

In this chapter, we will discuss some delicious keto recipes.

4.1. Muffins of Almond Butter

(Ready in 35 Mins, Serves: 12, Difficulty: Normal)

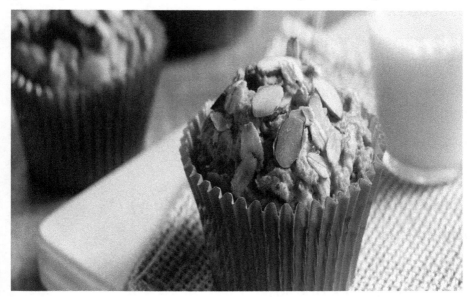

Ingredients:

- Four eggs
- 2 cups almond flour
- 1/4 tsp. salt
- 3/4 cup warm almond butter,
- 3/4 cup almond milk
- 1 cup powdered erythritol
- Two teaspoons baking powder

Instructions:

1. In a muffin cup, put the paper liners before the oven is preheated to 160 degrees Celsius.

2. Mix erythritol, almond meal, baking powder, and salt in a mixing bowl.

3. In another cup, mix the warm almond milk with the almond butter.

4. Drop some ingredients in a dry bowl till they are all combined.

5. In a ready cooker, sprinkle the flour and cook for 22-25 minutes until a clean knife is placed in the center.

6. Cool the bottle for five minutes to cool.

4.2. Breakfast Quesadilla

(Ready in 25 Mins, Serves: 4, Difficulty: Easy)

Ingredients:

- 4 eggs
- 1/4 cup (56 g) salsa
- 1/4 cup (30 g) low-fat Cheddar cheese, shredded
- 8 corn tortillas

Instructions:

1. When it is done, throw in the salsa, and whisk in the cheese to the very top. Sprinkle the oil on a few tortillas and then place a few pieces on an even number of the tortillas' edges.

2. Take the baking sheet. Divide the egg mixture between the tortillas, which is much more challenging. Oil-side up, cover the remaining tortillas. For 3 minutes or before the

golden brown heats up, grill the quesadillas on each side. Serve.

4.3. California Breakfast Sandwich

(Ready in 30 Mins, Serves: 6, Difficulty: Easy)

Ingredients:

- 1/2 a cup (90 g) chopped tomato
- 1/2 a cup (60 g) grated Cheddar cheese
- Six whole-wheat English muffins
- 2 ounces (55 g) mushrooms, sliced
- One avocado, sliced
- 6 eggs
- 3/4 cup (120 g) chopped onion
- 1 tbsp. unsalted butter

Instructions:

Beat the eggs together. Brown onion in a large oven-proof or high-sided skillet until clear. It's safe and tidy. Chop up avocado, tomatoes, and champagne onion blend and stir. Blend together. Proofread the attached work. Quickly cook until it's almost cooked. Add the salt, vinegar, and cheese. Spoon with English toasted muffins.

4.4. Stromboli Keto

(Ready in 45 Mins, Serves: 4, Difficulty: Normal)

Ingredients:

- 4 oz. ham
- 4 oz. cheddar cheese

- Salt and pepper
- 4 tbsp. almond flour
- 1¼ cup shredded mozzarella cheese
- 1 tsp. Italian seasoning
- 3 tbsp. coconut flour
- One egg

Instructions:

1. To avoid smoking, stir the mozzarella cheese in the microwave for 1 minute or so.

2. Apply each cup of the melted mozzarella cheese, mix the food, coconut fleece, pepper and salt together. A balanced equilibrium. Then add the eggs and blend again for a while after cooling off.

3. Place the mixture on the parchment pad and place the second layer above it. Through your hands or rolling pin, flatten it into a rectangle.

4. Remove the top sheet of paper and use a butter knife to draw diagonal lines towards the dough's middle. They can be cut one-half of the way on the one side. And cut diagonal points on the other side, too.

5. At the edge of the dough are alternate ham and cheese slices. Then fold on one side, and on the other side, cover the filling.

6. Bake for 15-20 minutes at 226°C; place it on a baking tray.

4.5. Cups of Meat-Lover Pizza

(Ready in 26 Mins, Serves: 12, Difficulty: Easy)

Ingredients:

- 24 pepperoni slices
- 1 cup cooked and crumbled bacon
- 12 tbsp. sugar-free pizza sauce
- 3 cups grated mozzarella cheese
- 12 deli ham slices
- 1 lb. bulk Italian sausage

Instructions

1. Preheat the oven to 375 F Celsius (190 degrees Celsius). Italian brown sausages, soaked in a saucepan of extra fat.

2. Cover the 12-cup ham slices with a muffin tin. Divide it into sausage cups, mozzarella cheese, pizza sauce, and pepperoni slots.

3. Bake for 10 mins at 375. Cook for 1 minute until the cheese pops and the meat tops show on the ends, until juicy.

4. Enjoy the muffin and put the pizza cups to avoid wetting them on paper towels. Uncover or cool down and heat up quickly in the toaster oven or microwave.

4.6. Chicken Keto Sandwich

(Ready in 30 Mins, Serves: 2, Difficulty: Normal)

Ingredients:

For the Bread:

- 3 oz. cream cheese
- ⅛ tsp. cream of tartar Salt
- Garlic powder
- Three eggs

For the Filling:

- 1 tbsp. mayonnaise
- Two slices bacon
- 3 oz. chicken
- 1 tsp. Sriracha
- 2 slices pepper jack cheese
- 2 grape tomatoes
- ¼ avocado

Instructions:

1. Divide the eggs into several cups. Add cream tartar, cinnamon, then beat to steep peaks in the egg whites.

2. In a different bowl, beat the cream cheese. In a white egg mixture, combine the mixture carefully.

3. Place the batter on paper and, like bread pieces, make little square shapes. Gloss over the garlic powder, then bake for 25 mins at 148°C.

4. As the bread bakes, cook the chicken and bacon in a saucepan and season to taste.

5. Remove from the oven and cool when the bread is finished for 10-15 mins. Then add mayo, Sriracha, tomatoes, and mashed avocado, and add fried chicken and bacon to your sandwich.

4.7. Keto Tuna Bites With Avocado

(Ready in 13 Mins, Serves: 8, Difficulty: Very Easy)

Ingredients:

- 10 oz. drained canned tuna
- ⅓ cup almond flour
- ½ cup coconut oil
- ¼ cup mayo
- 1 avocado
- ½ tsp. garlic powder
- ¼ tsp. onion powder
- ¼ cup parmesan cheese
- Salt and pepper

Instructions:

1. Both ingredients are mixed in a dish (excluding cocoa oil). Shape small balls of almond meal and fill them.

2. Fry them with coconut oil (it needs to be hot) in a medium-hot pan until browned on all sides.

4.8. Green Keto Salad

(Ready in 10 Mins, Serves: 1, Difficulty: Easy)

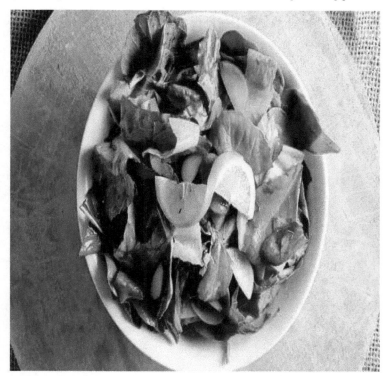

Ingredients:

- 100 g mixed lettuce
- 200 g cucumber
- 2 stalks celery
- 1 tbsp. olive oil
- Salt as per choice
- 1 tsp white wine vinegar or lemon juice

Instructions:

1. With your hands, rinse and cut the lettuce.

2. Cucumber and celery chop.

3. Combine all.

4. For the dressing, add vinegar, salt, and oil.

4.9. Breakfast Enchiladas

(Ready in 1 Hr., Serves: 8, Difficulty: Normal)

Ingredients:

- 12 ounces (340 g) ham, finely chopped
- Eight whole-wheat tortillas
- 4 eggs
- 1 tbsp. flour
- 1/4 tsp. garlic powder
- 1 tsp. Tabasco sauce
- 2 cups (300 g) chopped green bell pepper
- 1 cup (160 g) chopped onion
- 2 1/2 a cup (300 g) grated Cheddar cheese
- 2 cups (475 ml) skim milk
- 1/2 a cup (50 g) chopped scallions

Instructions:

1. Preheat the oven to 350 °F (180 °C). Combine the ham, scallions, bell pepper, tomatoes and cheese. Apply five teaspoons of the mixture to each tortilla and roll-up.

2. In a 30 x 18 x 5-cm (12 x 7 x 2-inch) non-stick pan. In a separate oven, beat together the eggs, milk, garlic, and Tabasco. Cook for 30 minutes with foil, then show the last 10 minutes.

Tip: Serve with a sour cream dollop, salsa, and slices of avocado.

4.10. Keto Mixed Berry Smoothie Recipe

(Ready in 5 Mins, Serves: 4, Difficulty: Easy)

Ingredients:

- 2 scoops Vanilla Collagen
- 1 cup of frozen Mixed Berries
- 2 cups Ice
- 1/4 cup Erythritol Powdered Monk Fruit
- 1 cup Unsweetened Coconut Milk Vanilla

Instructions

1. In a high-speed blender, combine all the ingredients.

2. Use or mix until smooth the "smoothie" setting.

4.11. Low-Carb Tropical Pink Smoothie

(Ready in 5 Mins, Serves: 1, Difficulty: Easy)

Ingredients: (makes 1 smoothie)

- $1/2$ small dragon fruit
- 1 tbsp. chia seeds
- 1 small wedge Gallia, Honeydew
- 1/2 a cup coconut milk *or* heavy whipping cream
- 1 scoop of whey protein powder (vanilla or plain), or gelatin or egg white powder.
- 3-6 drops extract of Stevia *or* other low-carb sweeteners
- 1/2 a cup water
- *Optional:* few ice cubes

Instructions

1. Monitor and place all the components smoothly in a mixer and pulse. Before or after combining this, you can apply the ice.

2. It is possible to include the fruit of a white or pink dragon. Serve.

4.12. Keto Peanut Butter Smoothie

(Ready in 1 Min, Serves: 1, Difficulty: Very Easy)

Ingredients:

- 1/2 a cup almond milk
- 1 tbsp. peanut butter

- 1 tbsp. cocoa powder
- 1-2 tbsp. peanut butter powdered
- 1/4 of avocado
- 1 serving liquid stevia
- 1/4 cup ice

Instructions

1. Add all the ingredients other than the ice and mix well in a food processor.

2. Apply enough milk to the smoothie for the ideal consistency. Add more ice or ground peanut butter to thin it out.

3. Serve it in a glass.

4.13. 5 Minute Keto Cookies & Cream Milkshake

(Ready in 5 Mins, Serves: 2, Difficulty: Easy)

Ingredients:

- $3/4$ cup heavy whipping cream or coconut milk
- Two large squares of grated dark chocolate
- **Optional:** frozen cubes of almond milk/ few ice cubes
- 1 cup unsweetened any nut or almond milk or seed milk
- 1 tsp vanilla powder or vanilla extract sugar-free
- 1-2 tsp Erythritol powdered, few drops of stevia
- $1/3$ cup walnuts or pecans chopped
- 2 tbsp. almond butter, (roasted or sunflower seed)
- 2 tbsp. coconut cream /whipped cream for garnishing

Instructions

1. Place in a blender, mix all the ingredients together (except topping). It is thicker as you blink. The ganache should be lit or topped with other ingredients.

2. Mix the whipped cream into the topping separately. Use 1/2 to 1 cup of milk for pounding. You should have whipped cream in the fridge for three days.

3. Pour some water into a bottle. Drizzle the nuts and butter leftover over the milk.

4.14. Keto Eggnog Smoothie

(Ready in 5 Mins, Serves: 1, Difficulty: Easy)

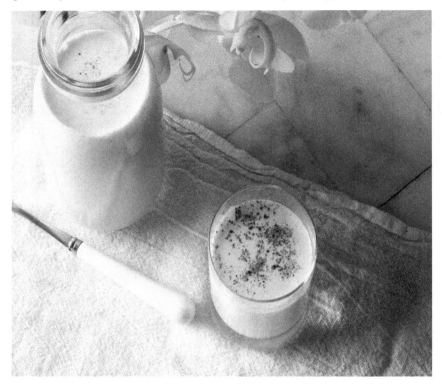

Ingredients:

- 1 Large Egg
- 1 tsp Erythritol
- 1/4 cup whipping cream (coconut cream for dairy-free)
- 1/2 tsp Cinnamon
- 4 Cloves ground approx. ¼ tsp
- 1 tsp Maple Syrup Sugar-Free (optional)

Instructions

In a blender, combine all the ingredients and mix fast for 30 seconds – 1 min.

4.15. Easy Keto Oreo Shake

(Ready in 5 Mins, Serves: 2, Difficulty: Easy)

Ingredients:

- 4 large eggs
- 2 tbsp. black cocoa powder or Dutch-process cocoa powder
- 1 1/2 cups unsweetened cashew milk, almond milk, or water 4 tbsp. roasted almond butter or Keto Butter
- 3 tbsp. Erythritol powdered or Swerve
- 1/4 cup whipping cream
- 1/4 tsp vanilla powder or 1/2 tsp vanilla extract (sugar-free)
- 1/2 a cup whipped cream for garnishing

•

Instructions

1. Place the frozen or cashew milk/almond milk in an ice cube tray and then freeze them. Under the right conditions (which means don't freeze the shake), miss this step and go on to the next.

2. Stir the cream in a tub of frozen milk. To produce ice cream, add ice cream to the warmed cream. Put some ova somewhere.

3. Apply the soaked nuts, sweetener, cacao powder, and vanilla to the dish. With macadamia, cocoa, cassava, and MCT, these oils are nice to use with MCT oil. Blend until smooth.

6. Apply more whipped cream before serving.

4.16. Keto Eggs Florentine

(Ready in 55 Mins, Serves: 4, Difficulty: Normal)

Ingredients:

- 1 tbsp. of white vinegar
- 1 Cup cleaned, the spinach leaves fresh
- 2 Tablespoons of Parmesan cheese, finely grated
- 2 Chickens
- 2 Eggs
- Ocean salt and chili to compare

Instructions:

1. Boil the spinach in a decent bowl or steam until it waves.

2. Sprinkle with the parmesan cheese to taste.

3. Break and put the bits on a tray. Place the tray on them.

4. Steam a hot water bath, add the vinegar and mix it in a whirlpool with a wooden spoon.

5. Place the egg in the center of the egg, turn the heat over and cover until set (3-4 minutes). Repeat for the second seed.

6. Put the spinach with the egg and drink.

4.17. Loaded Cauliflower (Low Carb, Keto)

(Ready in 20 Mins, Serves: 4, Difficulty: Easy)

Ingredients:

- 1 pound cauliflower

- 3 tablespoons butter
- 4 ounces of sour cream
- 1/4 tsp. garlic powder
- 1 cup cheddar cheese, grated
- 2 slices bacon crumbled and cooked
- 2 tbsp. chives snipped
- pepper and salt to taste

Instructions

1. Chop or dice cauliflower and switch to a microwave-safe oven. Add two water teaspoons and cover with sticking film. Microwave for 5-10 minutes until thoroughly cooked and tender. Empty the excess water, give a minute or two to dry. If you want to strain the cooking water, steam up your cooling flora (or use hot water as normal.)

2. Add the cauliflower to the food processor. Pulse it until smooth and creamy. Mix in the sugar, garlic powder and sour cream. Press it in a cup, then scatter with more cheese, then mix it up. Add pepper and salt.

3. Add the leftover cheese, chives and bacon to the loaded cauliflower. Place the cauliflower under the grill for a few minutes in the microwave to melt the cheese.

4. Serve and enjoy.

4.18. Crispy Drumsticks

(Ready in 1 Hr. 5 Mins, Serves: 4, Difficulty: Normal)

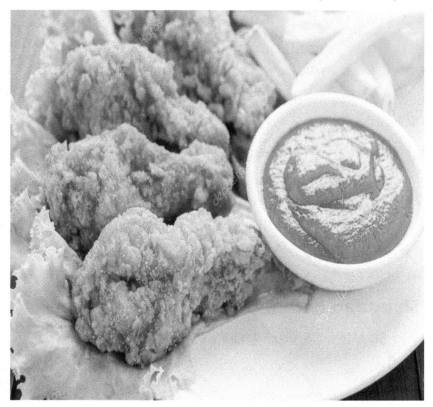

Ingredients:

- Dried thyme
- Olive oil
- 10 – 12 chicken drumsticks (preferably organic)
- Paprika
- Sea salt
- Black pepper

- 4 tbsp. Grass-fed butter or ghee, melted and divided

Instructions

1. Heat the oven to 375 F.

2. Line a rimmed baking sheet.

3. On the parchment paper, in a single sheet of holes between the drumsticks.

4. Mix 1/2 of the melted butter or ghee in olive oil with drumsticks.

5. Sprinkle on thyme and seasoning.

6. Turn it on for 30 minutes. Carefully empty the bottle and switch drumsticks over. When the drumsticks are cooling, produce a thyme and butter mixture again.

7. Return the pie for another 30 minutes (or until finely browned and externally baked).

4.18. Shredded Herbal Cattle

(Ready in 50 Mins, Serves: 4, Difficulty: Normal)

Ingredients:

- 2 tablespoons of rice wine
- 1 tbsp. of olive oil
- 1 pound leg,
- 2 Chipotle peppers in adobo sauce,
- 1 garlic clove chopped,
- Mature tomatoes, peeled and pureed
- 1 yellow onion
- 1/2 tbsp. chopped fresh Mustard

- 1 cup of dried basil
- 1 cup of dried marjoram
- 1/4 cut into strips beef
- 2 medium shaped chipotles crushed
- 1 cup beef bone broth
- Table salt and ground black pepper,
- Parsley, 2 spoonful's of new chives, finely chopped

Instructions:

In an oven, steam the oil in a medium to high heat. Continuously cook beef for six to seven minutes. Add all the ingredients to the beef. Heat and cook for 40 minutes; add the remaining to a moderate-low heat. Then tear the meat, have it.

4.19. Nilaga Filipino Soup

(Ready in 45 Mins, Serves: 4, Difficulty: Normal)

Ingredients:

- 1 Tsp. butter
- 1 tbsp. patis (fish sauce)
- 1 pound of pork ribs, boneless and 1 shallot thinly sliced bits,
- Split 2 garlic cloves, chopped 1 (1/2) "slice of fresh ginger, 1 cup chopped
- 1 cup of fresh tomatoes,
- 1 cup pureed "Corn."
- Cauliflower

- salt and green chili pepper, to taste

Instructions:

1. Melt the butter in a bowl over medium to high heat. Heat the pork ribs for 5-6 minutes on both sides. Stir in the shallot, the garlic and the ginger. Add extra ingredients.

2. Cook, sealed, for 30 to 35 mins. Serve in different containers and remain together.

4.20. Lemon Mahi-Mahi Garlicky

(Ready in 30 Mins, Serves: 4, Difficulty: Normal)

Ingredients:

- Kosher salt
- 4 (4-oz.) mahi-mahi fillets
- Ground black pepper
- 1 lb. asparagus
- 2 tbsp. extra-virgin olive oil,
- 1 lemon
- juice of 1 lemon and zest also
- 3 cloves garlic
- ¼ tsp. of crushed red pepper flakes
- 3 tbsp. butter, divided
- 1 tbsp. freshly parsley chopped, and more for garnish

Instructions:

1. Melt one tbsp. Cook some butter in a large saucepan, then add oil. Season with salt and black pepper. Mahia,

add, sauté. Cook for 5 minutes on each side. Transfer to a dish.

2. Apply one tbsp. of oil for the casserole. Cook for 4 minutes and add the spawn. Season with salt and pepper on a pan.

3. Heat butter to the skillet. Add garlic and pepper flakes and simmer until fragrant. Then add lemon zest, juice, and Persil. Break the mahi-mahi into smaller pieces, then add asparagus and sauce.

4. Garnish before consuming.

Conclusions:

An important element to note is eating a great combination of lean meat, greens, and unprocessed carbs. The most efficient way to eat a balanced diet is simply adhering to whole foods, mainly because it is a healthy solution. It is crucial to understand that it is impossible to complete a ketogenic diet.

If you're a woman over 50, you may be far more interested in weight loss. Many women experience decreased metabolism at this age at a rate of about 50 calories per day. It can be incredibly hard to control weight gain by slowing the metabolism combined with less activity, muscle degradation and the potential for greater cravings. Many food options can help women over 50 lose weight and maintain healthy habits, but the keto diet has recently been one of the most popular.

KETO FOR WOMEN OVER 50

Your Essential Guide to Lose Weight, Feel Younger and Live a Healthy Lifestyle After 50.

By Jason Smith

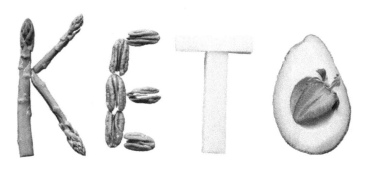

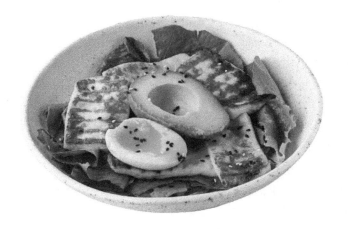

© **Copyright 2021 by (Jason Smith) - All rights reserved.**

This document is geared towards providing exact and reliable information in regards to the topic and issue covered. The publication is sold with the idea that the publisher is not required to render accounting, officially permitted or otherwise qualified services. If advice is necessary, legal or professional, a practiced individual in the profession should be ordered from a Declaration of Principles, which was accepted and approved equally by a Committee of the American Bar Association and a Committee of Publishers and Associations.

In no way is it legal to reproduce, duplicate, or transmit any part of this document in either electronic means or printed format. Recording of this publication is strictly prohibited, and any storage of this document is not allowed unless with written permission from the publisher. All rights reserved.

The information provided herein is stated to be truthful and consistent, in that any liability, in terms of inattention or otherwise, by any usage or abuse of any policies, processes, or directions contained within is the solitary and utter responsibility of the recipient reader. Under no circumstances will any legal responsibility or blame be held against the publisher for reparation, damages, or monetary loss due to the information herein, either directly or indirectly.

Respective authors own all copyrights not held by the publisher.

The information herein is offered for informational purposes solely and is universal as so. The presentation of the information is without a contract or any type of guarantee assurance.

The trademarks used are without any consent, and the publication of the trademark is without permission or backing by the trademark owner. This book's trademarks and brands are for clarifying purposes only and owners owned themselves, not affiliated with this document.

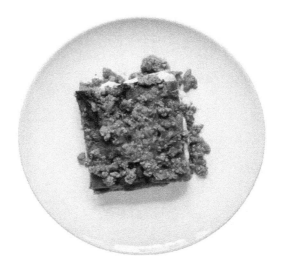

Introduction

Amongst living in what is considered a 'technologically advanced' 21st century, the hectic nature of day to day life often causes man to disregard the important factors that allow us to function the way we do; specifically our internal health. According to recent statistics, it is acknowledged that over 50% of employment is digitalized therefore justifying the ideology that obesity is a grave issue due to the lack of physical movement and interaction man has. Although a workout method may be suggested, it is of no use unless supported alongside a corresponding diet which would ensure that any fat is burnt properly and efficiently- This is something websites won't tell you.

Nowadays, it is fairly common to see the craze of salads doing wonders for the body; flat stomachs, idealistic bodies, sound perfect right? Although it has its benefits, such as providing nutrients to the body to stimulate powerful antioxidants in the blood- it does very little to reduce body mass. After years of research to find a diet plan that not only brings about good eating habits but also solves this issue equally as well, man has bought about a concept known as the "keto diet."In reality, theconcept was based around issues such as cancers, epilepsy, and Alzheimer's, and it was believed that keto wondered enabled the prevention of cells from gaining their energy from glucose (blood sugar); however, over time, many who had used this prog took notice of the weight loss advantages during participation, therefore,labeling this diet as what we now know to be a 'weight loss prog.'

Alongside the benefit of eating well, this diet is believed to encourage a regular and orderly eating schedule, which proves to be challenging in this day and age. However, normally our bodies would use our carbohydrate stores to provide the service of breaking down fats and play a role as a provider of energy. Still, in this case, the lack of carbohydrate intake due to this diet would force our bodies to extract energy from fat stores, which is a system known as 'Ketosis.'

Keto is most suited to those over 50 specifically because that is a period where women undergo menopause in which women experience symptoms such as hormonal changes and a loss of appetite, and weight loss. Keto is believed to relieve mostmenopause symptoms due to its high fat and very low carb diet. However, during that period, it is also common to see a fluctuation in insulin levels. Keto is believed to help its sensitivity ensure a more controlled blood sugar level.

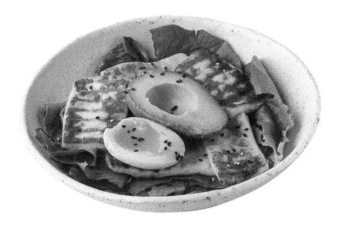

It helps the body more effectively burn its fat reserves. The ketogenic diet or keto diet involves removing carbohydrates from your diet and increasing fats. An eating plan that focuses on foods with lots of healthy fats, sufficient quantities of protein, and very few carbohydrates is a keto diet. The purpose is to promote more calories from fat than from carbohydrates. By depleting the body of its sugar stores, the diet operates. It will start to break down fat molecules for energy as a result. It contributes to the formation of molecules called ketones that the body uses for fuel. It may also cause weight loss as the body burns fat. The current study has shown that ketogenic diets are good for general health and weight loss.

1.1 How Ketogenic Diet Works?

Imagine your body as a car to understand why you could burn fat faster on a keto diet or be in ketosis. Your body breaks down food for energy into glucose: glucose is the petrol of your body. What happens when the body doesn't have enough glucose to use? Your car does not run without fuel in any situation. Fortunately, it doesn't happen in your body as well. You have the replacement fuel known as ketones, created by your liver from fat that brings your body into a ketosis state. You reduce carbohydrates and protein on a keto diet;it suggests eating a diet high in fat. Insufficient protein or carbohydrates means you don't have a ton of glucose for food.The backup fuel is used by your body, turning the fat you consume and body fat into ketones.

You burn fat for food, literally

You still manufacture ketones. But if you consume a ketogenic diet, glucose is replaced by ketones as the dominant fuel for your body, and you get into ketosis. It moves from glucose to ketones for days or weeks, and controlling it is also equally difficult. Also, tiny quantities of carbohydrates or extra protein will prevent ketosis from being preserved by your body.

1.2 What is Ketosis?

Ketosis is a metabolic condition in which the body uses fat and ketones rather than glucose as the main energy source (sugar). In your liver, as required for nutrition, glucose is stored and released. After all, after carb intake has been exceptionally low for one to 2 days, this glucose supply becomes depleted. The brain needs an adequate supply of fuel to function continuously, but the mechanism of 'gluconeogenesis' is not enough. That is where the liver produces glucose from the amino acids found within the ingested proteins.

1. The Ketosis process provides the body, specifically the brain, with an alternate source of energy. The body rapidly forms ketones during ketosis. Ketones, also known as ketone bodies, are formed exclusively from fat already present in your liver, eaten, and fat from your own body. Beta-hydroxybutyrate (BHB), acetoacetate, and acetone are the primary forms of ketone species.

2. Ketones are formed daily in the liver when consuming a higher-carb diet. It normally occurs often overnight while sleeping but in small numbers. During this, glucose and insulin levels are forced to decrease; however, the liver is on a carb-restricted diet, pushing to increase its ketone output to supply energy to the brain efficiently.

3. Until your blood crosses a certain ketone level, you are assumed to have nutritional ketosis. The 'edge' of nutritional ketosis is known to have a minimum of 0.5 mmol/L of BHBB.

4. While both fasting and a keto diet are useful, it will become obvious that a keto diet is sustainable over long periods. Besides, individuals should adopt easily finally.

1.3. Ketosis vs. ketoacidosis

Ketosis and ketoacidosis are both have a different concept, but they sound identical. The word 'ketoacidosis,' a form of 1 DM complication, refers to diabetic ketoacidosis (DKA). It is an extremely life-threatening disease that leads to a dangerously high level of ketones and blood glucose. For ketosis and ketoacidosis, as well as ketone, development takes place. It is known that ketosis is typically stable, while ketoacidosis can be life-threatening.

This blend makes the blood extremely acidic, directly targetingsensory organs' functioning in the body, such as the liver and kidneys. If this is the case, it is of the highest concern that it is handled. It can occur very quickly with DKA. In just 24 hours, it has the potential to expand. For those with type 1 diabetes whose bodies lack insulin, it is most prevalent. Many things could be caused by DKA, which is similar to illness, poor nutrition, or not taking a proper insulin dose. Many with type 2 diabetes with little or no development of insulin in their body are at risk of developing DKA.

Ketosis is a metabolic mechanism that starts when the body is on a low carbohydrate diet. After this, ketone bodies are formed by the liver. In ketosis, the ketone body's level rises to 8 mmol/l without causing changes to the pH value. The ketone bodies' level is forced to rise to 20 mmol/l during ketoacidosis, resulting in reduced PH levels. Both ketoacidosis and ketosis, therefore, contain ketones but have distinct efficiencies.

1.4. What are ketone bodies?

When there is an insulin deficiency in the blood, different chemicals are produced by the body. Instead of using glucose, internal fat is also allowed to break down as an energy supplier (sugar). All ketone species considered toxic acid chemicals are acetone, acetoacetate, and beta-hydroxybutyrate. They move through the blood and into the urine. Another way in which the body can get rid of acetone in the lungs (respiration). Ketosis is when ketone bodies are found in the blood, and urine containing ketone bodies is ketonuria.

The production house for liver ketones will manufacture ketone molecules at about 185 gs per day. Acetoacetate is a subform of liver-assembled ketones, whereas beta-hydroxybutyrate is the predominant blood circulating ketone molecules. After their formation, these are combined with acetyl coenzyme A (CoA) and join the 'Krebs cycle.' The Krebs cycle is considered a part of the metabolic pathway that uses oxygen to burn fuel to generate energy in organisms' breathing.

It is where they are used to produce energy molecules.

1.5. Types of Ketogenic Diets

The Keto Diet allows low carbohydrates and high fats to be consumed. Consumers are prohibited from buying candy, processed foods, grain and vegetable products. If one succeeds in implementing the exact delineated diet plan, all those health benefits enjoyed by those who have adopted the keto diet before can certainly be enjoyed.

1. The Ketogenic Regular Diet, or SKD

Proteins, fats, and carbohydrates are primarily the foundation of a ketogenic diet. Although the concentration of carbohydrates is between 5 and 10 percent, the protein concentration in keto diets fluctuates between 15 and 20 percent. That of fat in keto diets is up to 75 percent. However, it would help if you concentrated on incorporating fat-rich meals and snacks into the diet plan while preparing your meals to frame a keto diet since, under a keto diet, you need to eat 150 gs of fat per day. Besides, the concentration of carbohydrates in diet foods must be kept as low as possible such that the daily intake limit of carbohydrates, which is 50 gs, cannot be exceeded.

2. The Ketogenic Targeted Diet, or TKDD

The Intended Ketogenic Diet micronutrient ratio comprises 10-15 percent of carbohydrates, 60-70 percent of fat, and 20 percent of protein. Athletes who often need to eat carbohydrates before or during a workout typically follow this diet. Unlike the regular keto diet strategy, high carbohydrates can be eaten in conjunction with the Planned Ketogenic Diet.

3. The Ketogenic Cyclic Diet, or CKD

Targeted Ketogenic diet macronutrient ratio is 5-10 percent of carbohydrates, 75 percent of fat, and 15-20 percent of protein when on keto days; otherwise, 50 percent of carbohydrates, 25 percent of protein, and 25 percent of fat are composed of the macronutrient throughout off 'days.' The main goal of the Targeted Ketogenic Diet is to provide relief for keto dieters to turn on and off from ketosis while enjoying the diet simultaneously

4. The TKD or High-Protein Ketogenic Diet

The High-Protein Ketogenic Diet's macronutrient ratio is 5-10 percent carbohydrates, 60-65 percent fat, and 30 percent protein. It is recommended that those who aspire to opt for this kind of diet eat 120 gs of protein in tandem with 130 gs of fat daily. Most people are drawn towards this type of Keto diet due to a higher concentration of proteins and limited fats than other Keto diets.

Keto is a diet for weight loss. Low-carb keto diets, however, offer women in their 50s some significant additional benefits. Those advantages include:

1.   Reduced body fat

A lot of diets claim weight loss, but the weight is just water in many cases. Keto improves the burning of fat and has better outcomes than most of the other diets. Keto also targets abdominal fat preferentially, appropriately called visceral fat,

In women who are over 50, abdominal fat begins to increase. It increases the risk of stroke, cardiac arrest, and heart failure. Abdominal fat deposition is mainly due to the hormonal changes associated with menopause.

2.   Increased sensitivity to insulin

Carbs are digested and converted into glucose. When eating carbohydrates, your body releases the hormone insulin to ferry glucose into your liver and muscles. However, with age, the body's sensitivity to insulin decreases, meaning that the glucose is more likely to be converted into and processed as fat, contributing to weight gain.

Low carb diets increase insulin sensitivity. It ensures that the few carbs that you eat will not turn into fat. Increased insulin sensitivity also helps to regulate the levels of blood glucose. Low blood glucose levels are inextricably related to better overall health and a decreased risk of type 2 diabetes.

3.   Extent brain function

Menopausal women also encounter things like memory loss, mood swings, and difficulty focusing. It can also make them suffer from depression and anxiety. It's because estrogen levels, the primary female sex hormone, decrease during menopause, affecting the amount of glucose that enters your brain.

The keto diet gives your brain an additional source of fuel; ketones. On ketones and a low-carb diet, the brain functions better. Far less popular are problems like mood swings and memory loss.

A decreased risk of many neurological disorders is also associated with the keto diet, including Alzheimer's disease and Parkinson's disease, all of which are more common in people over 50 years of age.

4. Inflammation reduced

The process of aging could be difficult on your body. Menopausal women experienced knee and hip pain and headaches, and other non-specific forms of pain in the 1950s.

Keto is a greater diet, and certain fats are very helpful for calming inflammation. Healthy anti-inflammatory fats that can form part of the keto diet include the following:

- Olive Oil
- For example, oily fish, sardines, tuna, and salmon
- Avocados and Avocado Oil
- Walnuts

By comparison, foods such as refined carbohydrates, sugar, and processed foods are all associated with increased inflammation. These foods do not constitute part of the keto.

5. Improved lipid profile in blood

When approaching their 50s, many women experience elevated triglyceride levels. It could be the epitome of heart attacks. However, Low carb diets have been proven to reduce triglycerides and LDL cholesterol while being high in fat, alongside increasing 'Healthy HDL cholesterol. These improvements are associated with better cardiovascular health and a decreased risk of heart disease.

6. Decreased Blood Pressure

Research shows that the blood pressure of women appears to be lower than that of men. However, as you reach your 50s, there's a possibility of it changing, and menopause begins to come into effect. A range of serious medical conditions such as heart failure, kidney disease, and stroke are all about high blood pressure; It has been shown that the low-carb keto diet improves blood pressure levels.

7. Increased mass of bones

Aged women are more vulnerable to bone loss, which will ultimately grow into osteoporosis if left uncontrolled and untreated (a medical disorder characterized by weak, fracture-prone bones). Keto removes nutrients that are normally able to interfere with the absorption of calcium. Another advantage of keto is that it, combined with lots of leafy green vegetables that are naturally high in calcium, will improve bone health and density.

8. Weight Sheds

Losing weight has become something close to an impossible challenge as a person gets older. This issue arises from a decline in metabolism rate with age, lack of exercise, healthy activity, and poor diet. However, as the metabolic rate rises and the burning of fats contained in the human body continues to be used, the Keto diet provides the opportunity to combat various problems.

9. Better Sleeping

Sleep disorders such as sleep apnea and insomnia are usually encountered by around 30 years old. An individual must switch to low carb and high fat keto diet to alleviate this and obtain deep sleep at night with additional energy to counteract these disorders.

1.6. What You Can Eat on a Keto Diet

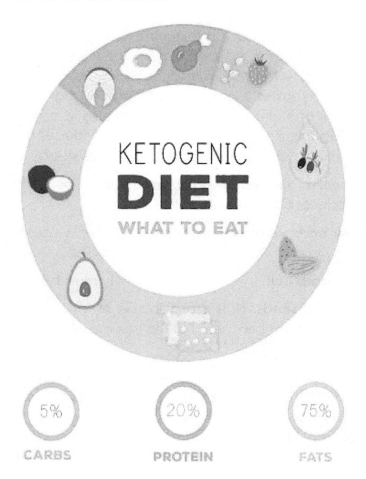

Keto-friendly fats

The largest aspect of a keto diet is to reduce your carb intake to 20-40 net gs per day to attain ketosis. To make sure you're still having the vitamins, minerals, and fiberin your body.

➢ Low carb vegetables

➢ Low carb fruits

➢ Poultry, meat, and eggs

➢ Cheese and other dairy products

➢ Seeds and nuts

1. **Poultry, meat, and eggs**: Unprocessed meat is preferred because it contains a minimum amount of carbs with no added carbs.In the keto diet, image findings are essential for eggs. One large egg contains less than 1 gm of carbohydrates, 5 gm of fat, and around 6 gm of protein in terms of nutrition. This nutrient profile is suitable for a ketogenic lifestyle. Egg white protein induces a sensation of fullness and keeps blood sugar levels steady.

2. **Cheese and other dairy products:** pick certain dairy products containing high fats.

3. **Low carb vegetables:** In the keto diet, vegetables that grow above the ground can be included.

4. **Low carb fruit:** the preferred quantity must be mild.

5. **Nut and seeds**: Nuts are a source of fat that is essential. But one must be careful of the volume of their intake.

Keto-friendly beverages: Low carb diets, including certain keto, have a mild diuretic effect, so be sure to drink at least 6 to 8 glasses of water daily, particularly during the induction process, to support your metabolism and normal body functions. The effect of not drinking enough water can be constipation, dizziness, and cravings. Sometimes, to ensure you get enough electrolytes, make sure you add extra salt to your diet. Try sipping your full-sodium broth on your food or adding a little extra salt.Up to 1/2 cup of decaffeinated or regular coffee and tea, herbal tea, sugar-free soy and almond milk, or any of these low-carb drinks are also allowed (without added barley or fruit sugar). Please pay close attention to your beverages, as they're still a big source of hidden sugars and carbohydrates without you knowing.

1.7. What You Can't Eat on the Keto Diet:

1. **Fruits**: are considered high in carbohydrates, so you might assumethat the candy of nature is off-limits on the popular high-fat, low-carbs, so almost all fruits are not permitted to eat in the keto diet.

2. **Legumes:** black beans, kidney beans,etc., are not allowed.

3. **Sweets:**Candy, sweets, cakes, buns, baked goods, tarts, pies, ice cream,cookies, custard, and puddings are not allowed in the keto diet.

4. **Rice:**A meal of no more than three ingredients

5. **Bread:** With a lower concentration of carbohydrates than usual bread

6. **Oatmeal:** With a drop in carb

7. **Pasta:** Getting little more than a recipe of two ingredients

8. **Cooking oil**: Choose from canola oil, soybean oil, grape oil, peanut oil, sesame oil, sunflower oil.

9. **Alcohol:**Keep it as dry as possible if you are going to spring for wine-the bottle should have less than 10g of sugar in its entirety

10. Bottled condiments: BBQ sauce, tomato sauce, certain salad dressings, and hot sauces that contain added sugar are bottled condiments that are not allowed.

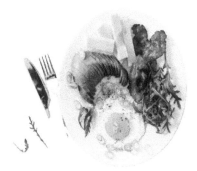

As you shift from adulthood to middle age, many physiological changes occur slowly over time in all body systems. These changes are life events, illness, genetics change, mood swings, and many other factors. According to a scientist, when a person crosses 50, both men and women start to gain 2-lb weight every year. It is most common in women because of their body system, like menopause, causing several hormonal changes in their body, which is weight gain.

Secondly, with aging, the metabolism of your body slows down with increasing age. Still, eating habits do not change, resulting in excess fat accumulation in your body, leading to weight gain. Secondly, your body's metabolism slows down with increasing age, but eating patterns do not change, resulting in excess fat accumulation in your body, leading to weight gain. It also moves forward about age in life, face muscle loss, skin thinning, stomach acidity reduction, and much more. Therefore, with age, by recognizing the variations occurring in the body, you have to start rethinking about eating behaviors to remain fit and safe. Before finalizing your meal schedule, you have to remember your daily workout routine.

People above 50 are less active than young people, so their calorie consumption should be decreased to minimize weight and foods rich in nutrients to remain healthy by consuming different foods to get the right and essential nutrients. Magnesium, omega-3 fatty acids, vitamin D, B12, calcium, iron, and potassium are essential components of older people's diet. Red blood cells responsible for oxygen delivery and brain health are created by vitamin B 12; calcium and vitamin D are essential for bone health. Iron is part of the balanced blood and circulatory system and several other complex benefits. It is also a necessary component of a diet and vitamins, proteins, fibers, and water. With aging, you have to keep the right amount of all these elements in your diet to stay away from diseases and stay healthy because as you get older, the body is unable to maintain the balance of these vitamins and other nutrients, so you can take supplements to support the body.

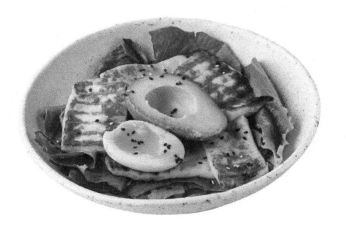

1. Change in metabolism

The metabolic rate decreases proportionately with the reduction in total protein tissue. At the very same time, total body fat typically increases with age. Aside from too many calories, lower metabolic rates may also explain this. People tend to increase weight and lose muscle as they get older. It explains why, as you get older, your metabolism will slow down. In general, since they have more body fat, heavier bones, and less body fat than females, men tend to have a faster metabolism.

2. Changes in bone

People, especially women after menopause, lose bone mass or density as they age. Calcium and other minerals are lost to the bones. Bones called vertebrae to make up the spine. A gel-like cushion between each bone is (called a disk)

They can break easily if the bones lose density. As time passes and people get aged, bone density changes. Bones absorb nutrients, water, and minerals during puberty and early adulthood.

3. Digestion Changes

This process often slows down as we age, and this may cause food to pass through the colon more slowly. More water is consumed from food waste as things slow down, which can cause constipation.

Aging may have dramatic effects on the digestive system's functions. Changes in hormone production and an alteration in smell and taste, one of these are decreased appetite. Dysphagia and reflux may result from physiological changes in pharyngeal skills and oesophageal motility. Also, aging can delay the immune system's response to antibodies being produced.

4. Sensory alterations

Odor and taste loss affect the food consumption and status of many older adults. It will not be eaten if no food smells or tastes appetizing.Stop eating vegetables until they are mushy. Try to roast or sauté fresh vegetables and toss them with garlic and olive oil until they are lightly fluffy.

Eat variety to meals by choosing foods with different flavored and colors. With dried cranberries and chopped nuts, coat the oatmeal. Add seeds, chickpeas, and crisp vegetables for salads. Start eating small meals more often throughout the day, instead of all three larger meals. It will help to increase your appetite and improve your senses.

5. Constipation and Dehydration

Among the most leading cause of chronic constipation is dehydration. Through your stomach to the large intestine, or colon, the food you consume finds its way. The broad intestine drains water from your food waste if you do not already have enough water in your body.

6. Teeth loss

Poorly fitting dentures will unintentionally alter eating habits due to chewing difficulties. Without important fresh fruits and vegetables, the result may be a sluggish, low-fiberdiet.As a way of preventing or slowing down the aging process, various items are advertised. Yet, there is no hard scientific evidence to prove that all these goods are healthy.

Instead, gerontologists (aging experts) suggest that people focus on staying healthy and well so that they can enjoy their favorite hobbies in middle age and beyond. Eating a balanced diet, which contains all the necessary nutrients for health, is a big part of a healthy lifestyle. Here are the main variables that, as you age, influence your nutritional health.

1. Needs for Calories

Our resting metabolic rate decreases as we grow older. It can lead to undesirable weight gain, which can increase the risk of some chronic diseases. As we age, this drop in metabolic rate is linked to the loss of lean body mass. To assist in reducing this effect:Increase your physical activity so that more calories are consumed.To strengthen your muscles and gain muscle mass, which increases your metabolic rate, start resistance training—incorporating whole grains, fruits and vegetables, lean protein, and non-fat or low-fat dairy improves your diet's consistency.

2. Proteins

For tissue development, repair, and maintenance, protein is essential. It's necessary to eat an adequate amount of protein each day, despite the need for fewer calories as we age. 45 to 60 gs are required by the average adult. Choose high-quality protein foods.

3. Dental health

Eighty percent of adult Americans are reported to have periodontal disease. Good practices in dental hygiene can help prevent it. As a result, foods such as fresh fruits, vegetables, and meat can be avoided. For the prevention of periodontal disease:

- Have dental tests and cleanings on an annual basis.
- During meals or after eating high-sugar food, brush your teeth.
- Floss periodically.

4. Taste

Sometimes, the senses of taste and smell are dulled by the aging process. Your sense of taste can also change with smoking and certain drugs. The protection of taste and smell:Keep hydrated; to completely taste the food, adequate saliva is required.

- Refrain from overusing the saltshaker.
- To boost the taste of food, use herbs and spices.

5. Antioxidant agents

There is no conclusive evidence that antioxidant supplements such as vitamin C or E can help prevent or postpone the aging process by avoiding chronic diseases. In reality, consuming foods rich in antioxidants (whole grains, fruits, and vegetables) and not taking supplements is beneficial. In your diet, include more of these

- To the Almonds
- Peppers from the Bell (especially red and orange)
- Blueberry
- Dark green vegetables with leaves
- Strawberry
- Tomatoes and Tomatoes

5. Vitamin D and Calcium

The bulk of the calcium in our bodies is in our bones. This mineral is needed for the nervous system's proper function, muscle contractions, and blood clotting. For the prevention and treatment of osteoporosis, sufficient calcium intake is crucial; vitamin D is important for calcium absorption. Dairy foods are also the best calcium source because the body can quickly absorb calcium in them.

The optimum amount of calcium for healthy adults is discussed by experts. Try to get all your calcium from food sources where possible. Except for fortified dairy products, vitamin D is not commonly present in foods. So you may need a supplement to take it. The body produces vitamin D from sunlight exposure, but people in northern climates do not get sufficient sun exposure to make adequate quantities of the vitamin in the winter. The new vitamin D intake guidelines suggest 600 IU for adults 19 to 70 years of age and 800 IU for those over 70.

6. Nutritional Supplements

If a person has a vitamin or mineral deficiency, health care practitioners usually do not prescribe dietary supplements. More research demonstrates that the best source of nutrients is food, not tablets or commercial beverages. Keep yourself in mind:

More is not necessarily better with vitamins; a multivitamin and mineral supplement should be everything you need to compensate for any shortfalls in your diet.

When eating a balanced diet, vitamin D and, in some cases, calcium is the only nutrients you need. There is insufficient evidence to encourage nutritional supplements with antioxidants.

7. Water

Sometimes, water is a forgotten nutrient. But for almost all bodily functions, having enough fluid is important. Approximately 1.5 to 2 liters or 48 to 64 ounces of fluid per day is required by healthy adults. As we age, the sense of thirst decreases, which leaves us susceptible to dehydration. Focus on non-diuretic beverages, such as decaffeinated foods, fruit juices, non-fat or low-fat milk, and water, of course.

 All these things come in a keto diet plan

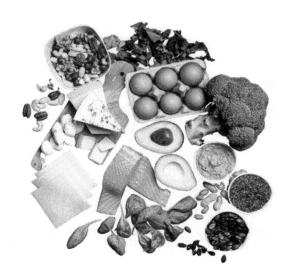

2.3. Is the keto diet good for women over 50?

One factor that never determines whether or notketo is right for you, but before assuming that keto is right for you, there are many factors involved.

Suppose you don't suffer from any significant health problems; in that case, a ketogenic diet will quench an enormous advantage, more precisely losing weight and getting rid of excess fat and obesity, the root cause of many. When eating vegetables, meat, and carbs, one must maintain equilibrium, as required. It is not easy to adapt and adhere to a ketogenic diet, as shown by many studies, so the best technique is to follow the balanced diet that suits you best and then stick to it. It is usually good to try new stuff, but one must think thousands of times before trying something new where there is a health danger.

The ketogenic diet is so genuine and successful that its consumers have consistently recorded its miraculous potency. Women record falling 11 lbs in seven days, up to 49 lbs in eight weeks, and almost 200+ lbs to their full limit so far, including in some instances, as reported.

2.4. How to start keto for women over 50

Keto is a simple diet, high carb diet to eating 50 gs of carbs or less per day is not always easy. It is just a mere difference in consumption and requires an adaptation in lifestyle that only exaggerates how much of a commitment this diet is. However, these minor changes deliver brilliant results and, in effect, are only the stepping stones to a healthier and sustainable life as it is guaranteed that these minuscule amendments will have a long-term effect not just physically but mentally too. Though at first, itmay seem intimidating, it does get much easier and understandable.

By following these instructions, make the transition into low carb keto dieting simpler.

1. Have a scheduled plan diet:

Keto is so specific from other diets that you cannot just jump in without doing your homework. Pick a start date and give yourself time to learn the ins and outs of low-carb dieting.

Learn more about what you can and can't eat. Spend this time gathering some low-carb instruments that may be useful, such as meal plans and recipes.

Also, tell your friends and family that you will 'go keto' and that your diet is about to change. Inform them to be supportive and agree that you won't eat bread, rice, pasta, etc.

2. Clear the unnecessary carbs out of your cupboards

Clean out any non-keto foods from your kitchen and refrigerator shortly before you begin your keto diet. You may think you can avoid temptation and not consume it, but the fact is that if you have easy access to high-carb foods, you are more likely to violate your diet.

However, don'teat any of these foods. The more carbohydrates you ingest, the harder and slower the transition to ketosis will be.

3. Using an app for food monitoring

Successful dieting with keto means restricting the consumption of carb to 50 gs a day or less. Using a food tracking app is the simplest and easiest way to lose weight and be your diet plan. Effective choices include good options,

It is an easy-to-use macro tracker; your meals can be fine-tuned to get the right carbohydrates, protein, and fat in your diet.

4. Realize that the first two weeks are the worst,

It's not always easy to get a keto, particularly for the first two weeks. Your body takes time to use all its onboard carb stores and instead make the transition to using ketones for energy. During this time, certain individuals experience adverse side effects, which as keto flu.

Although it is not serious and certainly you can feel unwell once the body completely reaches ketosis.

Popular symptoms of keto flu include:

- Headache
- Nausea
- Constipation
- Sleeplessness
- Fruity-odorous breath
- Increase in urination
- Tiredness
- Swings of mood
- Cravings

You are well on the way to being a machine for fat-burning. Your symptoms will fade soon, and they will fully pass within 1-2 weeks. Often, after they leave, and unless you cheat on your diet, only once can you ever suffer keto flu.

5. Don't cheat at all

Many diets allow you to take days off and even cheat by eating unhealthy foods from time to time. The keto diet is not either of those diets If you cheat on keto by consuming carbohydrates, you can push yourself out of ketosis to have to go through another bout of keto flu to get back on track.

Don't be tempted to trick keto. Long story short, it's just not worth it. Alternatively, in some types of therapy, reward your healthy eating habits. It's a nice idea to go to the movies, buy a new fitness suite, or treat yourself to a massage or beauty treatment. High carb food treats are not found in the ketogenic diet.

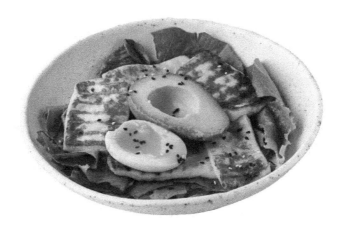

6. Think of using some well-picked supplements

Although you don't have to use supplements on the keto diet, for women over 50, they can make things simpler. Great choices include:

7. Ketones exogenous

Ketones from an external source are exogenous ketones. Taking exogenous ketone supplements will speed up burning fat, give you energy, keep your mind calm, and help alleviate many symptoms of keto flu. As drink blends and in capsules, exogenous ketones are available.

8. Triglycerides of the medium-chain

These specific fats are quickly and easily converted by MCTs, for short, into ketones. More ketones mean better fat burning and weight loss, more control, and fewerketo flu symptoms.

MCT supplements are used to make palm or coconut oil. However, coconut oil is the best and is also the most environmentally conscious choice. There are MCTs available as oils or in easy-to-mix powder form.

9. Electrolytes

In your urine, electrolytes are minerals that are excreted and even lost when you sweat.The keto diet raises urine production, which could mean that your body begins to run low on these vital substances. Symptoms of low electrolyte levels include headaches and muscle cramps. Electrolyte supplements supplement absent nutrients that can help prevent a number of symptoms of keto flu.

10. Treat keto as a way of life, not just a diet.

Most people think about a new diet; they just want it to be practiced for a few weeks. They figure that they will get through it until they have lost some weight and then go back to their previous eating habits. It eventually leads to weight loss, dubbed yoyo dieting by experts, followed by weight recovery. You will get even better keto outcomes if you accept low-carb dieting as a lifestyle choice and not a short-term fix. That way, you're not only going to lose weight, but you're also going to keep it off for good. Most of the benefits listed earlier in this chapter only refer to dieting on a low-carb basis. If you break your diet, lower blood pressure, improved cardiovascular health, reduced inflammation, and better bone health, you can say goodbye to such factors. If you break your diet, lower blood pressure, improved cardiovascular health, reduced inflammation, and better bone health, you can say goodbye to such factors. Keto is perfect for weight loss in your 50s, but it can be so much more than that as well. It can have a profound and substantial effect on any aspect of your welfare. After a few weeks or months, by reaching and quitting keto, do not give away those advantages. Instead, make a long-term commitment to low-carb diets. You will love the result if you do.

2.5. What makes keto-diet so powerful?

A ketogenic diet speeds up our body's metabolic response, which helps metabolically transform our body. If we do a detailed analysis, it will be discovered that one is persuaded to abstain from eating carbohydrates to the degree that ketosis is caused in one's body by following a keto diet. Several medical doctors reported that those patients who religiously followed the keto diet increased their fat-burning process by almost 900 percent. As a consequence, the hollowness caused by the internal burning of the fat causes them to shrink.

Another benefit of the keto diet is that it changes the human body's metabolism, accelerating its normal metabolism rate to about ten times. In deciding the metabolic rate, muscle tissues are used. A short study was carried out at a university in southern California, which demonstrated that they lose muscle tissue annually when women leap over 30 years of age. Besides, this phenomenon brings speed in tandem with time, some of them losing a substantial 20 percent of their muscles as they leap over the 60s, resulting in their metabolism slowing down. This lack of muscles causes a large chunk of their body mass, No need to worry because a keto diet is full of protein and healthy fats that trigger the revival of these missing muscles and provides them with an alternative. Thus, reviving metabolism and helping them sustain their healthy speed result from which, women will not suffer mass and health loss when they grow old.

Expediting metabolism is the key advantage that can be extracted from the keto diet. Still, certain secondary advantages of the keto diet include nourishing our body with satiety hormones and the like. Besides, many individuals feel dissatisfied adopting the diet plan in addition to providing a multitude of benefits. Most of them do not abstain from eating tasty items that catch their attention with carbohydrates. It is normally difficult to limit yourself from eating favorite meals and eating only the exact quantity of proteins, fats measured and carefully reduce the number of carbohydrates to 5 percent in our diet when consuming the number of meals three times a day. Many keto dieters claim that before getting completely beneficial from the keto diet, determining the diet plan requires math at a severely intimidating stage. This drastic calculation also results in a lack of motivation and satisfaction when following the diet, thereby leading most dieters to abandon their diet plan. However, as successful as keto is, many women are struggling with the diet. Many weight loss methods are too difficult to sustain long enough to build new behaviors, doctors explain. By decreasing carbohydrates, proteins, and fats to 5%, 25%, and 70%, respectively, the initial version of the keto diet asks to restrict macronutrients, and this measurement is very tiring and a hassle for most people, resulting in missing this calorie count most of the time

Fortunately, when preparing the diet, keto dieters have come across another way to get rid of the laborious math. The projected concept rests on keeping the diet plan easy in which one can bypass the traditional proposed keto diet and can forge their diet plan, and instructions on the diet plan could be obtained to help in this regard.

The Keto diet helps you get thin in no time, but it also helps minimize heart diseases. The keto diet also helps preserve the balance of cholesterol, preventing the usual defense and reversal of diabetes from artery damage three times. Besides, it is also beneficial to the brain because several repeated studies have shown that it significantly improves the dieter's memory and decreases arthritis discomfort.

2.6. A common problem

They envelop their frustrating tales and worst experience when trying to follow the keto diet, as reported by the number of physicians during the study that many patients give them emails. Doctors have often received an email from people who complained about the diet's ineffectiveness when saying they had diligently followed the diet plan. Still, sadly, however, they do not lose weight. Despite their urine showing that they are undergoing ketosis, some individuals complained that they are gaining weight instead of losing weight, causing them further anger. Let me clarify one explanation for this diet's ineffectiveness for women aged between 40 and 50 years. Do not worry if you are suffering from this anomaly because you are not alone. During the 1940s, many women in the United Kingdom and the United States had menopause. It does not matter which diet you adopt during this transition period; you will be gaining weight.

But it is advised that they should not worry, the best top ten tips for such individuals are carefully advised mentioned below but note if one out of many tips does not prove successful but must try because the last tip will be a practical one.

- **Get the proper quantity of protein**

Protein must be eaten to a moderate sustainable extent for weight loss. Moreover, It is proven by female physicians that women typically eat more protein than male partners; If a woman and her husband eat a protein-containing steak, she must consume it in more quantities than his husband.

Doctors had put forth an idea to tackle the confusing task of gcounting. A solution was A 'Mindful Week,' which was proposed by them. It requires the interpretation of the hunger and fullness principle. Doctors say that most of the Sapiens do not understand the basic notionand distinction between hunger and fullness. Discussing the real problem, doctors say that most women are not suffering because of menopause but because of their lack of appetite andfulfillment.

In the meantime, doctors' approach is limited to women experiencing menopause and is accessible to any woman over 30 who has decided to lose weight and improve health. Coming to a point, what is the week of mindfulness? It is a time commitment task during which, before recognizing that what is enough for her exceeds her original requirement, one has toobserve her hunger and fullness closely.

Let us consider a brief example of this method. Try eating two loaves of bread at breakfast, but you'll eat one instead of two today. After twenty mins, you will find either hungry or need one more leaf to kill your hunger. You will come to know the right amount of food to satisfy your appetite, following the same routine and sagaciously observing yourself. That will help you stop eating, which normally leads to gaining weight. But to have a healthy body with strong muscles, one should bear in mind that proteins are a vital part of a diet, so be very careful when cutting your protein intake.

- **Don't eat too much fat**

Since the keto diet is focused on high fats and low carbohydrates, for those who love to eat fats, this low carb keto diet is cheerful because it is included in every meal. Simultaneously, since fat is highly concentrated in the keto diet, one must abstain from consuming too much fat. According to experts, if you want to get rid of your weight, you must burn the body's fat. On the contrary, if one is persistent through his keto diet in eating fat and striving to burn fats accumulated in one's body, all his struggles will be wasted. Taking fats through the keto diet will replace those burned by the challenging efforts of one.

Doctors typically show that every new keto dieter is addicted to eating many carbohydrates in glucose, coffee, and whipping cream before adopting the keto diet. He recommended that they substitute these carbohydrates with high fats, and once they are completely removed from carbohydrates, they are then recommended to limit the fat limit. Due to its realistic use, the technique is proposed. It is much harder to get rid of the addictiveness of carbohydrates compared to that of fats. So it becomes easier for them to turn their diet from fat to keto-friendly food products without putting much effort when a person stops eating carbohydrates. Besides, a person typically begins to enjoy keto diet plans, producing more pleasant results.

When one gets rid of eating carbs' addictiveness and yet experiences a halt in weight loss, the volume of fat consumption must be considered. One will certainly figure out the real loophole causing this weight loss stall by analyzingits fat intake. In small steps, one must slowly cut back a min of coffee to stay relaxed while attempting to cut back some of the fat in one's diet to break the stall. In several situations, doctors remember that people complain about losing weight from the stall while saying that they strictly observe the keto diet but cannot produce the desired results. When doctors asked them to present their diet plan, which they were pursuing, it was discovered that by overdosing on coffee and whipped cream whose main constituent is fat, they were eating an abundance of fat. After recognizing their diet strategies, their respective doctor is recommended to cut back some of the fat they eat in coffee and whooping to break this stall and achieve the desired outcomes.

The good thing is that this technique does not place a total restriction on fat intake, but it only involves weight reduction by cutting fat before the stall breaks. The weight soon reaches the optimal amount; one can raise fat intake to whatever level one wants to eat.

- **Pay attention to the carb creep**

When an individual is thoroughly following the low carb, high fat keto diet, special care must be taken to avoid carbs' consumption. Carbs are often found in sauces, vegetables, nut snacks, and condiments. Often, carbohydrates will reach your diet without knowing by eating carelessly, so there is a huge risk of consuming carbs through sauces, fruits, nut snacks, and seasonings, which must be avoided by eating carefully.

Time and again, the same lesson is cited to emphasize the main factor to which people typically do not pay much attention, leading them to lose the efficacy of the keto diet. It is suggested that you need to revisit your current diet at the drop of a hat. There may be an abundance of carbs that have become unnoticeably part of your meal.

Nuts such as cashews and pistachios are difficult to overeat while having enough carbohydrates to lead to weight-loss stalling. Like, for example, pistachios, which contain around 21 gs of carbohydrates. Those people who avoid insulin can experience a ketosis stall for about three weeks if they eat food-containing carbohydrates. The dieter would certainly find a good outcome if the keto dieter carefully kept the amount of carbohydrate intake below 20 gs.

- **Cut the Alcohol Out**

Alcohol lovers are experiencing ketosis, and they are persuaded that they should have a few bottles of weekly wine time and time again following a low carb diet plan. But for them, it is bad news that alcohol overconsumption may lead to a weight-loss stall. However, if one comes to know that, while thoroughly pursuing one's keto diet schedule, one is not losing weight, one should doubt that alcohol intake is this stall. It would be wise to cut back all wine intake before the ketosis started again if caught in such a situation.

- **Stop eating sweets**

Many individuals are likely to use artificial flavors to feel relaxed when eating the keto diet. Even if these sweeteners, such as sucralose or aspartame, give one's meal the perfect taste, it may be equally disadvantageous for those who observe the keto diet. Typically, therefore, experts prohibit keto dieters from adding sweeteners to their diets. Experts do not clarify why one should avoid using sweeteners because of a lack of studies on this topic, but most agree with the decision.People who cut sweeteners from their diet lose weight easily.

- **Get enough sleep**

A proper night's sleep plummets with tension and cortisol. Cortisol is a stress hormone that induces an increase in abdominal fat when elevated. Owing to night sweats and hot flashes, women suffering from menopause still face a condition in which their sleeping routine is ruined. It is recommended for these women, who are involved in weight loss, to keep their primary focus on following their proper sleeping routine while going through the menopause era, keeping all stresses at bay. A bad sleeping pattern causes cortisol, a stress hormone linked to abdominal fat, while increasing the human body's weight.

For better sleep, tips include:

- ➤ Limit caffeine intake and stop drinking coffee
- ➤ Spend some time in the sunlight.
- ➤ Using eyeshades and earplugs to wear
- ➤ Try to restrict screen time before reaching the bed to stop the blue light (or if possible, use glasses that blocks blue light)
- ➤ Craft a suitable sleeping schedule and religiously execute it.
- ➤ It must be cool and dark in the sleeping room.
- ➤ Stop drinking before reaching the bed.
- • Stress Reduction

Weaning off all sorts of stresses that you are dealing with is vital. Stress often puts one's mental and physical health at an adverse risk.

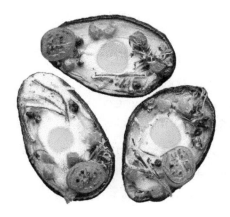

Below is a range of recipes recommended by nutritionists and experts to help get your diet started. Most require normal 'around the house' items to help get your breakfast, lunch, and dinner in full swing,

1) Bacon Breakfast Biscuit

Ingredients:

> ➢ 6 bacon slices (chopped).

> ➢ 3 large eggs

> ➢ 1 cup cheddar cheese (grated)

> ➢ 1 cup onion (chopped)

> ➢ 1 cup green peppers (chopped)

> ➢ ¾ cup almond flour

> ➢ 1 tsp baking powder

- ➢ ½ tsp salt
- ➢ ½ tsp pepper
- ➢ Cooking spray

Instructions:

1. Preheat the oven to 375 degrees C.

2. Spray the cooking spray with a large frying pan and fry the bacon until it is crisp and browned. Add the onions and peppers, cut the bacon and fry until tender.

3. Mix the almond flour, baking powder, salt, and pepper in a bowl until well mixed.

4. Whisk the eggs in a separate bowl and add half a cup of the cheese; add the mixture of eggs to the flour mixture and blend until well combined; whisk in the cooked bacon.

5. Line a baking tray with greaseproof paper; spoon to flatten 12 individual round biscuits slightly with the back of a spoon on the sticky mixture.

6. Sprinkle the remaining cheese over it and bake for 10 mins.

Nutritional Information:

- ➢ Total servings - 12 Per serving: (1 biscuit)
- ➢ Fat: 33g
- ➢ Carbohydrates: 4g
- ➢ Protein: 31g
- ➢ Calories: 451

2) Egg & Goats Cheese Medley

Ingredients:

- ➢ 8 large eggs
- ➢ 1 tomato (chopped)

- ➤ 2 oz goats' cheese
- ➤ 2 tbsp water
- ➤ ¼ cup mixed fresh herbs (chopped)
- ➤ 1 tbsp butter
- ➤ ½ tsp salt
- ➤ ¼ tsp black pepper

Instructions:

1. Whisk the eggs, salt, pepper, and water together.

2. Heat the butter in a large frying pan, add the egg mixture and cook for 2-3 mins, mix in the tomatoes and remove from the heat.

3. Fold the goat's cheese and herbs together.

Nutritional Information:

- ➤ Total servings - 4 Per serving
- ➤ Fat: 10g
- ➤ Carbohydrates: 2g
- ➤ Protein: 15g
- ➤ Calories: 249

3)   Nutty Cottage Cheese Fruit Mingle

Ingredients:

- ➤ ¾ cup cottage cheese
- ➤ ¼ cup frozen mixed berries
- ➤ 3 tbsp walnuts (chopped)
- ➤ 1 tsp flaxseed oil
- ➤ 1 tsp chia seeds.

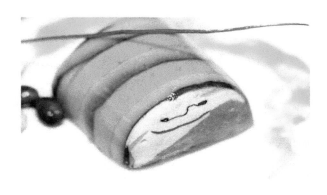

>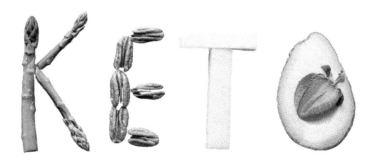

Instructions:

1. In a bowl, add the cottage cheese and drizzle it with flaxseed oil.

2. Sprinkle with the chia seeds and finish with walnuts and mixed berries.

Nutritional Information:

- ➤ Total servings - 1 Per serving
- ➤ Fat: 23g
- ➤ Carbohydrates: 11g
- ➤ Protein: 19g
- ➤ Calories: 312

4) Egg & Bacon Sandwich Twist

Ingredients:

- ➤ 4 bacon slices
- ➤ 3 large eggs
- ➤ 1 tomato (chopped)
- ➤ 1 spring onion (chopped)
- ➤ ¾ cup mozzarella
- ➤ ¾ cup cheddar cheese
- ➤ Cooking spray

Instructions:

1. Preheat the oven at 400 and line a baking tray with parchment paper.

2. Mix the cheese and spread it on the tray evenly, creating a circle—Bake for approximately 5 mins.

3. Spray with a cooking spray on a frying pan, fry the bacon until crispy and remove from the pan. Spray and scramble the eggs with a little more cooking spray.

4. On one half of the cheese circle, put the bacon and eggs: sprinkle on the tomato and onion.

5. Over the bacon and eggs, fold the cheese circle in half, press down firmly, and bake for 5 mins.

Nutritional Information:

- ➢ Total servings - 2 Per serving:
- ➢ Fat: 35g
- ➢ Carbohydrates: 5g
- ➢ Protein: 33g
- ➢ Calories: 445

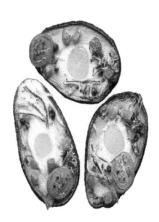

5) Chorizo & Egg Breakfast Buns

Ingredients:

- ➢ 12 eggs
- ➢ 6 oz cheddar cheese (grated)
- ➢ 5 oz chorizo (chopped)
- ➢ 2 spring onions (chopped)
- ➢ Salt and pepper

> Cooking spray

Instructions:

1. Preheat the oven to 350 and grease a large muffin tray.

2. Add the chorizo and onions to the bottom of each hole in the muffin tray.

3. Whisk the eggs, cheese, salt, and pepper together; pour the onions and chorizo on top.

4. Bake until done, for approximately 20-25 mins.

Nutritional information:

> Total servings - 6 Per serving: (2 buns)

> Fat: 27g

> Carbohydrates: 2g

> Protein: 23g

> Calories: 335

6) Loaded Avocado

Ingredients:

> 4 eggs

> 4 cherry tomatoes (chopped)

> 6 oz bacon (chopped)

> 2 avocados

> Cooking spray

Instructions:

1.Preheat the oven to 375.

2. Spray cooking spray onto a frying pan and fry the bacon until crispy.

3. Cut the avocados, remove the stone; to fit an egg, and scoop out enough flesh.

4. On a baking tray, put the avocados and crack an egg in each hole. Sprinkle the tomatoes over the eggs along with the bacon.

5. Bake for 20 mins until the eggs are cooked thoroughly.

Nutritional Information:

> ➢ Total servings - 2 Per serving:
> ➢ Fat: 73g
> ➢ Carbohydrates: 6g
> ➢ Protein: 25g
> ➢ Calories: 803

7) Coconut & Blueberry Porridge

Ingredients:

> ➢ 1 large egg
> ➢ ¼ cup blueberries
> ➢ 1 oz butter
> ➢ 1 tbsp coconut flour
> ➢ 4 tbsp coconut cream
> ➢ 1 pinch psyllium husk powder

Instructions:

1.In a cup, whisk the egg and stir in the psyllium husk and coconut flour.

2. Melt the butter on low heat and add the coconut milk. Combine the egg mixture slowly until it becomes thick and fluffy.

3. Add the blueberries.

Nutritional Information:

> ➢ Total servings - 1 Per serving:

- ➢ Fat: 50g
- ➢ Carbohydrates: 4g
- ➢ Protein: 10g
- ➢ Calories: 488

8) Sweet & Spicy Stuffed Peppers

Ingredients:

- ➢ 8 ounces Cream cheese
- ➢ 8 mini bell peppers
- ➢ 1 ounce's chorizo (chopped)
- ➢ 2 tbsp Olive oil for
- ➢ 1/2 tbsp Chipotle paste

Instructions:

1.Mix all ingredients until well combined.

2. Put the mixture of spoons into peppers.

Nutrition facts:

- ➢ Total servings - 4 Per serving
- ➢ Fat: 31
- ➢ Carbohydrates: 8g
- ➢ Protein: 8g
- ➢ Calories: 343

9) Cheesy Cauliflower Combo

Ingredients:

- ➢ Cauliflower 28 ounces (chopped)
- ➢ Broccoli 16 ounces (chopped)
- ➢ Cheddar cheese 8 ounces (grated)

- ➤ Cream cheese of 7 ounces
- ➤ 1 cup of cream thick
- ➤ Two ounces of butter
- ➤ 2 Tsp of powdered garlic

Instructions:

1.Boil the broccoli in a large saucepan until thoroughly cooked and tender.

2. Strain and leave the broccoli in a saucepan; add cream cheese, thick cream, butter, and powdered garlic.

3. Purée until smooth and creamy using a blender

4. Grease a large baking platter and add florets of cauliflower.

5. Pour over a mixture of creamy broccoli and top with cheese.

6. Cook until the cauliflower is tender and the cheese is golden, for 40-45 mins.

Nutrition Facts:

- ➤ Total servings - 6 Per serving
- ➤ Fat: 45g
- ➤ Carbohydrates: 11g
- ➤ Protein: 18g
- ➤ Calories: 5133

10) Avocado &Chili Crab Salad

Ingredients:

- ➤ 12 ounces of meat from crab (canned)
- ➤ 4 eggs of large size (boiled)

- ➤ 2 avocados
- ➤ 2 ounces baby Spinach
- ➤ 2 tbsps Olive oil
- ➤ 1/2 cup Mayonnaise
- ➤ 1/2 cup of cottage cheese.
- ➤ 1/2 tbsps of chili flakes

Instructions:

1.Slice the avocados and chop the boiled eggs into halves.

2. Drain the meat from the crab and stir in the chili flakes.

3. Place the eggs, avocado, mayonnaise, cottage cheese, crab meat, and spinach on a plate.

4. Drizzle the spinach with olive oil.

Nutritional details:

- ➤ Total Portions - 2 Per Portion
- ➤ Fat: 98g Fat:
- ➤ Carbohydrates: 7g
- ➤ 44g Protein
- ➤ 1097 Calories

11) Cheeky Cheesy Chips

Ingredients:

- ➤ Cheddar cheese 8 ounces (grated)
- ➤ Cheddar cheese 8 ounces (grated)
- ➤ Chili flakes with 1/2 tsp
- ➤ 1/2 tsp of paprika

Instructions:

1.Preheat the oven to 400.

2. Line a parchment paper baking tray and a cheese spoon into separate piles.

3. Sprinkle chili flakes and paprika with cheese piles and bake until fully melted and golden for 10 mins.

4. Allow to cool down.

Nutritional Information:

- ➢ Total servings - 4 Per serving
- ➢ Fat: 22g
- ➢ Carbohydrates: 2g
- ➢ Protein: 12g
- ➢ Calories: 229

12) Bacon & Halloumi Sausages

Ingredients:

- ➢ 8-ounce halloumi
- ➢ 6 ounces Bacon

Instructions:

1. Preheat the oven to 425.
2. Cut the halloumi into 10 chunks and wrap around each chunk with a slice of bacon.
3. Bake for 15-20 mins, turning until cooked through and golden brown occasionally.

Nutritional Information:

- ➢ Total servings - 2 Per serving
- ➢ Fat: 63g
- ➢ Carbohydrates: 4g
- ➢ Protein: 33g
- ➢ Calories: 703

Ingredients:

- ➤ Pork shoulder of 48 ounce
- ➤ 6 cloves of garlic
- ➤ 6 leaves of Iceberg lettuce
- ➤ 2 onions of red
- ➤ 3/4 cup of red wine
- ➤ 1/2 cup of olive oil
- ➤ 2 tbsps of cilantro (finely chopped)
- ➤ Salt of 1/2 tsp
- ➤ Ground cinnamon with 2 tsps
- ➤ 2 black pepper tsp
- ➤ Dried thyme with 2 tsps

Instructions:

1. Preheat the stove to 250.
2. Slice the onions into thin wedges and cut the garlic in half.
3. Add the remaining marinating ingredients. In a large ziplock bag, put the pork shoulder and pour in the marinade.
4. Seal the bag and put it in a big dish overnight, in refrigerate.
5. Place the pork and marinade in a large oven-proof dish, cover with a close-fitting lid.
6. Bake for 6-7 hours in the lower portion of the oven.
7. Pork is exceptionally tender to serve on top of lettuce leaves and take apart.

Nutritional Information:

- ➢ Total servings - 4 Per serving
- ➢ Fat: 92g
- ➢ Carbohydrates:11g
- ➢ Protein: 63g
- ➢ Calories: 1141

14) Pan-Seared Pork & Pepper

Ingredients:

- ➢ 10-ounce pork (cut into strips)
- ➢ 4-ounce butter
- ➢ 1 red pepper (chopped)
- ➢ 1 yellow pepper (chopped)
- ➢ 1 red onion (sliced)
- ➢ 1 tsp chili paste.

Instructions:

1. Heat butter in a pan on high heat and brown pork for 3 mins.
2. Add in remaining ingredients and fry until thoroughly cooked.

Nutritional Information:

- ➢ Total servings - 2 Per serving
- ➢ Fat: 79g
- ➢ Carbohydrates: 4g
- ➢ Protein: 29g
- ➢ Calories: 840

15) Zucchini & Sausage Stew

Ingredients:

- ➤ 16 ounces sausage
- ➤ Mozzarella 8 ounces (grated)
- ➤ Marinara sauce with 7 ounces
- ➤ 6 ounces of bacon (chopped)
- ➤ Cream cheese of 4 ounce
- ➤ 4 ounces of parmesan (grated)
- ➤ Two zucchinis (grated)
- ➤ For 2 eggs
- ➤ 1 of onions (finely chopped).

Instructions:

1. Preheat the oven to 400.
2. Mix until well combined: zucchinis, cream cheese, milk, parmesan, and 4 oz mozzarella.
3. For 18-20 mins, pour the mixture into an oven-proof dish and bake.
4. Cook the onions, sausage, and bacon in a large frying pan until cooked through.
5. Take the zucchini from the oven, spread it over the marinara sauce, and top it with the sausage mixture.
6. Top and bake for an additional 15 mins with the remaining mozzarella.

Nutritional Information:

- ➤ Total servings - 6 Per serving
- ➤ Fat: 59g
- ➤ Carbohydrates: 8g
- ➤ Protein: 33g

- ➤ Calories: 693

Ingredients:

- ➤ 16 ounces of beef mince.
- ➤ 14 ounces of tomatoes whole (canned)
- ➤ Spinach 7 ounces
- ➤ Mozzarella for 5 ounces
- ➤ Two ounces of butter
- ➤ ounces of parmesan (grated)
- ➤ For 1 egg
- ➤ Olive oil 3 tbsps
- ➤ tbsps of chives (chopped)
- ➤ 1 tsp salt
- ➤ 1 tsp of powdered garlic
- ➤ Onion powder of 1/2 tbsp
- ➤ Dried basil 1/2 tsp
- ➤ Black pepper, 1/2 tsp

Instructions

1. Mix the beef, parmesan, egg, and spices in a large bowl until well combined.
2. Make the blend into meatballs of walnut size.
3. In a frying pan, heat the oil and fry the meatballs until cooked and browned.
4. Turn down the heat and add the chives and tomatoes.
5. Allow 15-20 mins to simmer.

6. Melt the butter and fry the spinach for 2 mins in a separate frying pan and add to the meatballs.

7. On a serving plate, put the meatballs, tear up the mozzarella, and drip over the meatballs.

Nutritional Information:

➢ Total servings - 4 Per serving

➢ Fat: 51g

➢ Carbohydrates: 4g

➢ Protein: 40g

➢ Calories: 626

17) Salmon & Pistachio Hot Pot

Ingredients:

➢ 15-ounce fillets of salmon

➢ 10 ounces of cherry tomatoes

➢ 1/2 cup of green olives (pitted & chopped)

➢ 1/3 cup of pistachio nuts (chopped)

➢ 1/4 cup of olive oil

➢ 1/4 cup of fresh dill (chopped)

Instructions:

1. Preheat the oven to 350.

2. Mix the olives and pistachios along with a splash of olive oil until well blended.

3. In an oven-proof bowl, put the salmon fillets and spread the olive mixture around the dish. Place the tomatoes in a separate oven-proof dish and cover with olive oil.

4. Bake both for 15 mins and sprinkle them with dill until thoroughly cooked.

Nutritional Information:

- ➢ Total servings - 2 Per serving
- ➢ Fat: 69g
- ➢ Carbohydrates: 7g
- ➢ Protein: 48g
- ➢ Calories: 844

18) Chicken with Onion Mayo

Ingredients:

- ➢ 16-ounce breast of chicken
- ➢ 7 ounces of green cabbage (chopped)
- ➢ 1/2 cup of mayonnaise
- ➢ 1/2 of red onion (finely sliced)
- ➢ 1 tbsp Olive oil
- ➢ Spray for cooking.

Instructions:

1. Cook the chicken until thoroughly cooked in a large frying pan sprinkled with cooking spray. Mix the onions and mayonnaise.

2. Place the chopped cabbage and drizzle with olive oil in the middle of the serving plate.

3. Place the chicken on top of the cabbage gently and put onion mayonnaise on the side.

Nutritional Information:

- ➢ Total servings - 2 Per serving
- ➢ Fat: 93g
- ➢ Carbohydrates: 7g
- ➢ Protein: 47g

> Calories: 1039

Ingredients:

- A minced beef of 14 ounces
- 9 ounces of cherry tomatoes (halved)
- 3 onions chopped)
- 3 carrots (chopped)
- 3 cloves of garlic (grated)
- 1/2 head of cauliflower (cut into florets)
- 1/4 cup of olive oil.

Instructions:

1. Preheat the furnace to 350.
2. Boil the water in a wide pan and add the cauliflower; cook until tender.
3. In a frying pan, add a little olive oil and cook until the carrots, onion, and garlic are cooked through.
4. Add the minced beef to the frying pan and cook until the tomatoes are browned.
5. Pour the mixture of beef into an oven-proof dish.
6. Add cauliflower and a little olive oil in a bowl, mash cauliflower until creamy and smooth. Spoon the cauliflower mixture over the beef and bake until golden brown for 20 mins.

Nutritional Information:

- Total servings - 6 Per serving
- Fat: 20g
- Carbohydrates: 9g

- ➤ Protein: 15g
- ➤ Calories: 270

20) Aromatic Spinach & Cheese Curry

Ingredients:

- ➤ Spinach of 14 ounces
- ➤ 7 ounces halloumi (cubed)
- ➤ Curry paste of 3 tbsps
- ➤ Olive oil for 2 tbsps
- ➤ 1 tbsp of cumin seed
- ➤ 1 slice of black pepper.

Instructions:

1. Mix the olive oil and curry paste in a large bowl; stir in the cubed halloumi.

2. Pour the mixture into a frying pan and cook until the cheese starts to melt for 5-6 mins. Toast the cumin seeds in a separate frying pan until they start to smoke; add some olive oil and spinach, fry until cooked, and season with pepper.

3. Place the spinach and top with cheese on a serving plate.

Nutritional Information:

- ➤ Total servings - 2 Per serving
- ➤ Fat: 42g
- ➤ Carbohydrates: 9g
- ➤ Protein: 29g
- ➤ Calories: 519

Ingredients:

- ➤ 2-ounce margarine
- ➤ 4 tbsp coconut flour
- ➤ 1-ounce walnuts
- ➤ ½ tbsp ground cinnamon
- ➤ One sharp apple
- ➤ ¾ cup substantial whipping cream
- ➤ 0.75 tbsp vanilla concentrate

Instructions:

1. Combine coconut, nuts, margarine, vanilla concentrate, and cinnamon to frame a batter.
2. Placed scaled-down bits of apple on a container lubed with oil.
3. Pour batter over the bits of apple.
4. Bake in a preheated stove at 350 degrees for 15 mins.
5. Mix half tbsp vanilla concentrate and whipping cream and beat until it gets soft.
6. Serve top heated apples with whipping cream and serve.

Nutritional Fact:

- ➤ Total Time: 20 mins
- ➤ Serving: 4
- ➤ Calories 340 kcal
- ➤ Proteins 3 g
- ➤ Carbohydrates 6 g

> Cholesterol 85 g

> Fat 33 g

Ingredients:

> 2 tbsp all that bagel preparing

> 1 cup cheddar

> 2eggs

> 1/2 cup parmesan cheddar ground

Instructions:

1. Whisk egg and cheddar in a bowl.

2. Pour in a doughnut container lubed with oil.

3. Drizzle flavoring over the egg blend.

4. Bake in a preheated stove at 375 degrees for 20 mins.

Nutritional Fact:

> Time: 17 mins

> Serving: 6

> Calories 218 kcal

> Proteins 14 g

> Carbohydrates 3 g

> Cholesterol 104 g

> Fat 16 g

Ingredients:

> Four pieces of cut bacon

> 1/4 tbsp dark pepper

- ➤ 1/2 hacked onion
- ➤ 1/2 tbsp stew powder
- ➤ 1/2 tbsp spread
- ➤ One diced avocado
- ➤ 1/2 tbsp cumin
- ➤ 1/4 tbsp salt
- ➤ Four eggs
- ➤ 8 ounce cut radishes
- ➤ 1.25 cups hacked chime peppers
- ➤ 1/4 cup packed cilantro

Instructions:

1. In a huge, measured skillet, cook bacon.
2. Take out the bacon when it becomes firm and saved.
3. Chop the bacon when they get chill off.
4. In a similar container, over medium fire, cook onion and radish for five mins.
5. Add half tbsp of oil whenever required.
6. Add hacked ringer pepper and cook for the following four mins.
7. Add salt, stew powder, and dark pepper.
8. Make very nearly four spaces by siding the veggies and pour the egg in those spaces.
9. Cover the dish and cook for five mins. Mood killer the fire
10. Sprinkle hacked bacon, avocado, and cilantro and serve.

Nutritional Fact:

- ➤ Total Time: 35 mins

- ➢ Serving: 4
- ➢ Calories 253 kcal
- ➢ Proteins 12.5 g
- ➢ Carbohydrates 11 g
- ➢ Cholesterol 72 g
- ➢ Fat 18.5 g

24) Keto Banana Pancakes

Ingredients:

- ➢ 1 tbsp cinnamon
- ➢ Two bananas
- ➢ ½ tbsp preparing pop
- ➢ Four eggs

Instructions:

1. Combine all the fixings in a bowl.
2. In a dish, dissolve spread over medium warmth.
3. Place a spoonful blend in the container and cook for a little from the two sides while covering the dish.
4. Serve with coconut cream.

Nutritional Fact:

- ➢ Total Time: 15 mins
- ➢ Serving: 4
- ➢ Calories 117 kcal
- ➢ Proteins 6 g
- ➢ Carbohydrates 14 g
- ➢ Cholesterol 164 g

➢ Fat 4 g

Ingredients:

➢ Two cuts of lettuce

➢ Four cut tomato

➢ Four cuts cooked of bacon

➢ Black pepper to taste

➢ 1 tbsp mayonnaise

➢ salt to taste

Instructions:

1. Take each lettuce in turn and spot it over a plain surface.

2. Spread mayonnaise over lettuce leaves, place two bacon cuts, and tomato.

3. Drizzle pepper and salt over tomatoes and wrap the leave and serve.

Nutritional Fact:

➢ Total Time: 15 mins

➢ Serving: 2

➢ Calories 336 kcal

➢ Proteins 8 g

➢ Carbohydrates 2.7 g

➢ Cholesterol 42.8 g

➢ Fat 32.7 g

26) Cream cheese scrambled eggs

Ingredients:

➢ 2 tbsp spread

- ➤ Two eggs
- ➤ 1 tbsp whipping cream
- ➤ One squeeze pepper
- ➤ 2 tbsp cream cheddar
- ➤ One squeeze salt

Instructions:

1. Whisk cream, pepper, eggs, and salt in a bowl.
2. Melt spread in a container and pour egg blend in it.
3. Mix cream cheddar.
4. When the egg blend begins to set from the edges, overlay it to permit the fluid under the stream.
5. Cook until the blend is set as wanted and serve.

Nutritional Fact:

- ➤ Calories 181 kcal
- ➤ Proteins 8 g
- ➤ Carbohydrates 1.3 g
- ➤ Cholesterol 0 g
- ➤ Fat 16 g

27) Keto coconut porridge

Ingredients:

- ➤ One squeeze of psyllium husk powder
- ➤ 4 tbsp coconut cream
- ➤ 1 egg
- ➤ 1 squeeze salt
- ➤ 1 tbsp coconut flour
- ➤ 1oz spread

Instructions:

1. Whisk coconut flour, salt, egg, and husk powder.

2. In a dish, liquefy coconut cream and margarine.

3. Slowly pour egg blend with consistent mixing to get a thick combination.

4. Take out in a serving dish.

5. With coconut milk, serve the porridge.

Nutritional Fact:

➤ Total Time: 10 mins

➤ Serving: 1

➤ Calories 481 kcal

➤ Proteins 9 g

➤ Carbohydrates 4 g

➤ Cholesterol 30 g

➤ Fat 48 g

28) Keto Sausage with Creamy Basil Sauce

Ingredients:

➤ 8-ounce mozzarella

➤ 3 lb. Italian chicken wiener

➤ ¼ cup basil pesto

➤ 8-ounce cream cheddar

➤ ¼ cup hefty cream

Instructions:

1. Place wiener in a lubed dish and prepare for 30 mins in a preheated broiler at 400 degrees.

2. Mix well hefty cream, pesto, and cream cheddar.

3. Pour the rich sauce over the prepared hotdog.

4. Spread mozzarella cheddar over the top and prepare for an additional ten mins.

Nutritional Fact:

➢ Total Time: 45 mins

➢ Serving: 8

➢ Calories 436 kcal

➢ Proteins 28 g

➢ Carbohydrates 2 g

➢ Cholesterol 146g

➢ Fat 46 g

29) Cheesy Keto garlic bread

Ingredients:

➢ Bread with garlic

➢ 1/2 tsp of salt

➢ 3 eggs

➢ 3 tbsps powder of psyllium husk

➢ 1 tsp powder for baking

➢ 1 tsp of onion powder

➢ 1 cup of mozzarella cheese grated

➢ 1/2 cup of flour of coconut

➢ 1 tsp powder of garlic

➢ 1 cup of hot water

➢ 1 tsp of oregano

➢ 1 cup of flour of almond

Butter on Garlic

- ➤ 1/2 chopped cloves of garlic
- ➤ 1/4 cup of butter
- ➤ 1/2 tbsp of oregano
- ➤ 1/2 tsp of salt
- ➤ tbsps Parmesan shredded cheese

Instructions:

1. Combine half a tbsp of minced garlic, half a tbsp of oregano, half a tbsp of salt, half a cup of butter, and two tbsps of cheese.

2. Mix all the garlic bread ingredients, except water and egg, in a mixing bowl.

3. Mix the flour with the eggs and mix well to make the crumbled dough.

4. Then add water and blend to get a smooth, firm dough.

5. Set it in a baking dish and roll the dough into a sheet.

6. Bake at 350 degrees for 20 mins in a preheated oven.

7. Brush the top of the bread after baking with a garlic butter mixture and sprinkle the mozzarella cheese over the bread.

8. Bake once again and serve for 20 mins.

Nutritional Fact:

- ➤ Total Time: 60 mins
- ➤ Serving: 10 slices
- ➤ Calories 197 kcal
- ➤ Proteins 9 g
- ➤ Carbohydrates 8.5 g
- ➤ Cholesterol 72 g
- ➤ Fat 15 g

Ingredients:

- 3 tbsps of sesame seeds
- 2 cups of almond flour
- 2 tbsps olive oil
- 1/4 tsp of salt
- 7 eggs
- 2 tbsps of chia seeds
- 1/2 tsp of xanthan gum
- 1/2 cup of butter
- 1 tsp powder for baking

Instructions:

1. Whisk the eggs together in a cup.

2. Chia seeds, baking powder, xanthan gum, sugar, salt, oil, and almond flour are whisked into the egg mixture using an electric beater.

3. Pour the batter and drizzle the sesame seeds into the baking pan.

4. Bake at 355 degrees for 40 mins in a preheated oven.

5. Slice the bread after cooling and store it in the fridge.

Nutritional Fact:

- Total Time: 50 mins
- Serving: 16
- Calories 175 kcal
- Proteins 6 g
- Carbohydrates 4 g

- ➤ Cholesterol 106 g
- ➤ Fat 16 g

Ingredients:

- ➤ Marinade
- ➤ 1 tsp cumin powder
- ➤ 1 tbsp lemon juice
- ➤ Chicken 900 gs
- ➤ 2 tsp of turmeric powdered
- ➤ 1 cup of yogurt
- ➤ Salt to taste
- ➤ 1 tbsp of garam masala
- ➤ Butter Sauce
- ➤ One chopped jalapeno pepper
- ➤ 2 tbsps of almond flour
- ➤ One Onion Chopped
- ➤ 60 gs of butter
- ➤ 1 tbsp of grated ginger
- ➤ 1 cup of heavy cream
- ➤ 1/4 tsp cinnamon powder
- ➤ 1tbsp vegetable oil
- ➤ 14 oz of sliced tomatoes
- ➤ 1/2 cup of chicken broth
- ➤ Three chopped cloves of garlic
- ➤ Salt to taste

Instructions:

1. Combine the garam masala, salt, lemon juice, cumin, pepper, yogurt, and turmeric in a mixing bowl.

2. In a tub, add the chicken pieces and mix well so that the chicken is well coated.

3. For better results, put the bowl in the refrigerator overnight.

4. Heat the oil in a pan and add the butter.

5. Stir in the onions when the butter is melted and cook for 4 mins.

6. Mix the onion with the cinnamon, ginger, garlic, and cumin seeds and cook for an additional four mins.

7. Mix the salt, tomatoes, and chilies and cook for ten mins when the onions turn orange.

8. Mix the onion mixture with the chicken, including the marinade.

9. Add the broth after five mins of cooking, then bring it to a boil.

10. The pan is sealed and simmered for the next 15 mins.

11. Mix the almond flour and cream and simmer for another 15 mins.

12. By using salt and pepper, change the flavor accordingly.

13. For garnishing, use cilantro leaves.

Nutritional Fact:

➢ Total time: 60 mins

➢ Serving: 6

➢ Calories 367 kcal

➢ Proteins 36 gs

- ➤ Carbohydrates 7 gs
- ➤ Cholesterol 146 g
- ➤ Fat 22 gs

Ingredients:

- ➤ 1/4 cup of almond flour
- ➤ 1/2 tsps puree of garlic
- ➤ 12 oz hearts of artichoke
- ➤ 1 Tbsp of lemon zest
- ➤ 1/4 cup of green onions chopped
- ➤ 1/4 Tsp dried oregano
- ➤ 2 Tbsps of olive oil
- ➤ 1/3 cup Pecorino-Romano shredded cheese
- ➤ Salting to taste
- ➤ 1/3 cup of Parmesan cheese grated
- ➤ 2 tbsps lemon juice
- ➤ 1/2 tsp dried thyme
- ➤ Black pepper to taste
- ➤ 1/3 cup of mayonnaise

Instructions:

1. Next, make the same-size slices of artichoke hearts.

2. Using oil to grease the baking tray.

3. Using a baking tray to create a single layer of artichoke hearts.

4. Drizzle over the top of the artichoke hearts with chopped onions, black pepper and salt.

5. Combine the shredded parmesan cheese, dried herbs, almond flour and pecorino romano cheese in a mixing bowl to create a fine, smooth paste.

6. Mix the lemon juice with the garlic puree, zest and mayonnaise.

7. Take half a cup of the mixture of cheese and blend in the garlic puree mixture.

8. Brush the mixture with the cheese over the artichoke hearts.

9. Cover with foil on the baking sheet.

10. Bake at 325 degrees for 30 mins in a preheated oven.

11. Spread the remaining cheese mixture over the artichoke hearts after 30 mins and bake at 375 degrees for another 25 mins.

12. Dish the artichoke hearts out and serve the dish while they are sweet.

Nutritional Fact:

- ➢ Total Time: 70 mins
- ➢ Serving: 4
- ➢ Calories 295 kcal;
- ➢ Proteins 9 g
- ➢ Carbohydrates 15 g
- ➢ Cholesterol 22 g
- ➢ Fat 24 g

33) Chicken green curry

Ingredients:

- ➢ 150 g of beansprouts
- ➢ Two chopped stalks of lemongrass

- ➢ 1 tbsp groundnut oil
- ➢ 1 tsp Thai sauce for fish
- ➢ Two Zest of Lemons
- ➢ 1/2 cup of chicken broth
- ➢ 700 g breast of chicken
- ➢ One diced clove of garlic
- ➢ Coriander as required for garnishing
- ➢ 200 g of green beans
- ➢ 1 tbsp lemon juice
- ➢ 13 oz of coconut milk
- ➢ Thai green curry paste 2 tbsp

Instructions:

1. In a pan, fry bite-sized chicken bits.

2. Add the curry paste, garlic, lemongrass, and lime zest when the chicken pieces have turned orange.

3. Cook and add chicken stock, coconut milk, and lime juice for 3 mins.

4. Cover it and let it simmer on a low flame for 10 mins.

5. Mix the green peas after 10 mins of simmering, then cook.

6. Combine the bean sprouts after two mins.

7. Switch off the flame after cooking for one min.

8. Garnish with coriander and serve with cauliflower rice.

Nutritional Fact:

- ➢ Total Time: 20 mins
- ➢ Serving: 4
- ➢ Calories 452 kcal

- ➤ Proteins 61 g
- ➤ Carbohydrates 7.5 g
- ➤ Cholesterol 158 g
- ➤ Fat 17 g

34) Keto beef kabobs

Ingredients:

Marinade

- ➤ 1 tsp powder of garlic
- ➤ 1 tsp of black pepper
- ➤ 2 tbsps olive oil
- ➤ 1 tsp of salt
- ➤ 1 tbsp of oregano
- ➤ 3 tbsps of vinegar (red wine)
- ➤ 1 tsp of onion powder
- ➤ 1 tsp of sauce Worcestershire

Cooking Steak

- ➤ 85 g of red, green, and yellow bell pepper for each
- ➤ Cube-shaped 1.5 lb. sirloin steaks
- ➤ 113 g red onion sliced
- ➤ 8 mushrooms

Instructions:

1. Combine the pepper, salt, oregano, garlic powder, Worcestershire sauce, vinegar, powdered onion and olive oil in a mixing bowl.

2. To get better results, add steak pieces and put them overnight in the fridge.

3. Thread beef alongside vegetables on a stick.

4. On medium heat, put a grill and heat the oil inside.

5. Over the grill, place threaded kabobs.

6. Brush the marinade over the kabobs regularly and continue changing the sides until both sides are fried.

Nutritional Fact:

- ➤ Total Time: 50 mins
- ➤ Serving: 8 kabobs
- ➤ Calories 168 kcal
- ➤ Proteins 19 g
- ➤ Carbohydrates 4 g
- ➤ Cholesterol 51 g
- ➤ Fat 7 g

35) Super simple braised red cabbage

Ingredients:

- ➤ 1/2 tsp ghee
- ➤ 2 tsp of erythritol (optional)
- ➤ 1/4 cup vinegar for cider (apple)
- ➤ One red onion sliced
- ➤ Black pepper to taste
- ➤ 2 tbsps of water
- ➤ Salt to taste
- ➤ 1/1 lb. of red cabbage chopped

Instructions:

1. Heat the ghee over a medium flame in a pan.

2. Sauté the onion for three mins in a pan.

3. Incorporate salt, erythritol, vinegar, chopped cabbage, pepper, and simmer for 7 mins.

4. Cover the pan after seven mins and cook on a low flame for 60 mins.

5. It can be kept in an air-tight container for up to five days.

Nutritional Fact:

- Total Time: 75 mins
- Serving: 4
- Calories 117 kcal
- Proteins 2 g
- Carbohydrates 7.9 g
- Cholesterol 10 g
- Fat 7.8 g

36) Labneh cheese ball

Ingredients:

- Flavored Oil
- 6 garlic cloves chopped
- 1/2 cup of olive oil
- 2 red chilies (dried)

For Labneh

- 3 tbsps of dill and mint chopped
- 1 tsp of salt
- 4- glasses of Greek yogurt

Instructions:

Flavoured Oil

1. Mix the chilies and garlic in a jar in a medium-sized mason jar.

2. To the pot, apply the olive oil and hold it for three days.

Labneh

1. To drain, pour yogurt into a strainer. Let it drain by leaving it in the refrigerator for three days.

2. Connect salt to the drained yogurt after three days and make small balls out of it.

3. Mix the finely chopped dill and mint in a dish.

4. Roll the yogurt balls to coat the balls in the dill and mint mixture.

5. Drop balls with flavored oil in a mason jar. When needed, add more olive oil.

6. Balls have to be completely dipped in grease.

7. Serve yogurt balls with vegetables or pita chips or bread on a serving plate.

Nutritional Fact:

- ➢ Total Time: 14 mins
- ➢ Serving: 6
- ➢ Calories 250 kcal
- ➢ Proteins 14 g
- ➢ Carbohydrates 7 g
- ➢ Cholesterol 0 g
- ➢ Fat 18 g

37) Keto Caesar salad

Ingredients:

- ➢ 2 tbsp of chopped anchovy
- ➢ 1 tbsp of mustard (Dijon)

- ➤ 1/4 cheese of parmesan (grated)
- ➤ Salt to taste
- ➤ Black pepper to taste
- ➤ One diced clove of garlic
- ➤ 1/2 cup of mayonnaise
- ➤ 1/2 lemon juice and zest
- ➤ Salad
- ➤ 7 oz of chopped lettuce
- ➤ 12 oz. breast of chicken
- ➤ 3 oz of bacon
- ➤ 1/2 cup of parmesan cheese (grated)
- ➤ 1 tbsp of olive oil
- ➤ Salt to taste
- ➤ Black pepper to taste

Instructions:

1. Mix the mustard, salt, lemon juice, cheese, anchovies, black pepper, garlic, lemon zest, and mayonnaise in an immersion mixer. Store it aside.

2. Place the chicken pieces and sprinkle them with black pepper, oil, and salt in a baking pan, greased with oil.

3. Bake the chicken for 20 mins at 350 degrees in a preheated oven.

4. Take a pan and fry the bacon in it while the chicken is in the oven.

5. Place some lettuce in a serving bowl.

6. Place the bacon and baked chicken pieces over the lettuce leaves and pour the pieces over the prepared dressing.

7. Garnish with and serve the grated cheese.

Nutritional Fact:

- ➢ Total Time: 35 mins
- ➢ Serving: 3
- ➢ Calories 997 kcal
- ➢ Proteins 71 g
- ➢ Carbohydrates 5 g
- ➢ Cholesterol 0g
- ➢ Fat 77 g

38) Chicken, spinach, and bacon salad

Ingredients:

- ➢ 1 cup of keto dressing ranch
- ➢ 150 g of spinach
- ➢ 1 cup of mushrooms chopped
- ➢ 5 Slices of Bacon
- ➢ 2 Breast Chicken
- ➢ 1 diced clove of garlic
- ➢ Basil as needed
- ➢ 4 tomatoes sun-dried
- ➢ 2 tsps olive oil

Instructions:

1. Heat the oil in a pan.
2. Garlic for cooking chicken until the chicken turns orange.
3. On a pan, take out the chicken bits.
4. Cook the bacon in the same pan.

5. In a dish, mix the bacon, chicken, mushrooms, spinach, and basil.

6. Spread the spinach into a serving dish and place the mixture of chicken and bacon over the spinach.

7. Drizzle the mixture with sun-dried tomatoes.

8. Store in the refrigerator for two days and use ranch dressing to serve.

Nutritional Fact:

- ➢ Total Time: 20 mins
- ➢ Serving: 3
- ➢ Calories 553 kcal
- ➢ Proteins 35 g
- ➢ Carbohydrates 3.3 g
- ➢ Cholesterol 0 g
- ➢ Fat 3.7 g

39) Keto broccoli salad

Ingredients:

- ➢ 2 tbsps of vinegar (apple cider)
- ➢ 1/2 cup of pumpkin seeds
- ➢ 8 sliced broccoli cups
- ➢ 1/2 lb. of bacon cooked and shredded
- ➢ 3/4 cup of mayonnaise
- ➢ 1/4 cup of red onion chopped
- ➢ Salt to taste
- ➢ 4 ounces of cheddar cheese
- ➢ Black pepper to taste

➤ 5 tsps of erythritol

Instructions:

1. Combine erythritol in a bowl with vinegar and mayonnaise. To get a smooth dressing combination, blend well.

2. Combine the pumpkin seeds, broccoli, cheese, and onion in a mixing bowl.

3. Pour the dressing into a bowl of broccoli mix.

4. Place the bowl in the refrigerator to cool and let the dressing and salad settle for three hours.

5. After drizzling with black pepper and salt, serve.

Nutritional Fact:

➤ Total Time: 10 mins

➤ Serving: 10

➤ Calories 266 kcal

➤ Proteins 8 g

➤ Carbohydrates 4 g

➤ Cholesterol 0 g

➤ Fat 25 g

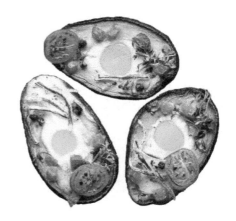

40) Keto Fried Eggs with Kale and Pork

Ingredients:

- ½ lbs kale
- 1 ounces cranberries
- 6-ounce pork belly smoked
- 1-ounce walnuts
- Salt to taste
- 3-ounce butter
- Four large eggs
- Pepper to taste

Instructions:

1. First sliced kale after trimming.
2. In a pan, melt butter (0.75 ounces) and add kale.

3. Cook on medium flame.

4. When kale edges turned brown, take out kale on a plate and set aside.

5. Add and cook pork in the same pan.

6. When pork becomes crispy, reduce the flame to low and add cooked kale walnuts and cranberries.

7. After the pan's content gets warm, then empty the pan in a serving bowl.

8. In the same pan, crack eggs separately in the remaining butter. Sprinkle black pepper and salt and fry to the desired level.

9. Put cooked eggs in a bowl with cooked pork, nuts, and kale and serve.

Nutritional Fact:

➤ Total Time: 20 mins

➤ Serving: 2

➤ Calories 1033 kcal

➤ Proteins 26 g

➤ Carbohydrates 8 g

➤ Cholesterol 141 g

➤ Fat 99 g

41) Halloumi Cheese Fingers

Ingredients:

➤ ½ tbsp olive oil

➤ tsps lemon juice

➤ 6 ounces halloumi cheese

➤ Pepper to taste

➢ ¼ tsps oregano

Instructions:

1. With a medium flame, heat olive oil in a saucepan.

2. Cook halloumi cheese for 2 mins or until turned brown.

3.Drizzle oregano, lemon juice, and black pepper and serve.

Nutritional Fact:

➢ Total Time: 10 mins

➢ Serving: 2

➢ Calories 299 kcal

➢ Proteins 18 gs

➢ Carbohydrates 3 gs

➢ Cholesterol 64 milligs

➢ Fat 25 gs

42) Mexican frittata

Ingredients:

➢ 1 tsp olive oil

➢ ¼ cup milk

➢ One sliced bell pepper (red)

➢ ½ salsa

➢ Two whole eggs

➢ One chopped white onion

➢ Four egg whites

➢ ½ tsp salt

➢ 1 tsp black pepper

➢ Pinch of cumin

Instructions:

1. , heat olive oil on medium in a skillet flame, sauté onion, and red bell pepper for about five mins.

2. In a mixing bowl, whisk eggs, egg white, milk, salt, cumin, and black pepper.

3. In a baking dish, place a stir-fried onion mixture.

4. Add egg mixture over onion and bell pepper mixture.

5. in a preheated oven at 350 degrees for 30 mins.

6. Make slices of the frittata and serve with salsa.

Nutritional Fact:

- ➤ Total Time: 50 mins
- ➤ Serving: 2
- ➤ Calories 202 kcal
- ➤ Proteins 17 g
- ➤ Carbohydrates 16 g
- ➤ Cholesterol 188 g
- ➤ Fat 8.5 g

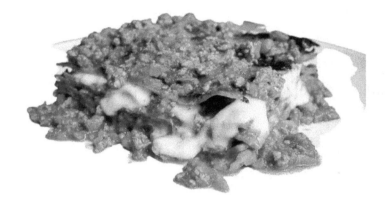

Ingredients:

- ➢ 4 ounces pancetta diced
- ➢ 5 eggs
- ➢ 1/4 tsp salt to taste
- ➢ 1/2 cup chopped onion
- ➢ 1/2 tsp chopped garlic
- ➢ 1/2 cup chopped tomato
- ➢ 1/4 cup almond milk
- ➢ 1/2 cup chopped oregano
- ➢ 1/2 cup chopped basil
- ➢ 1 cup tomato sauce

- ➢ Black pepper to taste
- ➢ Red pepper flakes for garnishing
- ➢ 2/3 cup grated parmesan cheese
- ➢ Oregano for garnishing

Instructions:

1. In a pan, add onion and pancetta in a skillet and sauté for two mins.

2. Turn off the flame

3. In a mixing bowl, add cheese and milk and whisk them well.

4. Add tomato, herbs, garlic, tomato sauce, black pepper, salt, and mix.

5. Add tomato mixture in skillet with pancetta and onion.

6. Placing eggs in the pan makes a small space using a spatula by moving the mixture aside.

7. Break eggs and pour them in spaces created in a mixture: one egg in each space.

8. Put some cheese on the upper surface.

9. For 15 mins ake in a preheated oven at 425 degrees

10. Use flakes and parsley to garnish and serve.

Nutritional Fact:

- ➢ Total Time: 28 mins
- ➢ Serving: 4
- ➢ Calories 207 kcal
- ➢ Proteins 14 g
- ➢ Carbohydrates 6 g
- ➢ Cholesterol 204 g
- ➢ Fat 14.4 gs

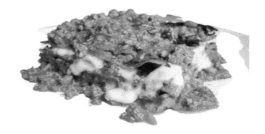

44) Halloumi Cheese Fingers

Ingredients:

- ½ tbsp olive oil
- 2 tsps lemon juice
- 6-ounce halloumi cheese
- Pepper to taste
- ¼ tsp oregano

Instructions:

1. With the gas on a medium flame, heat olive oil in a saucepan.

2. Cook halloumi cheese for 2 mins or until turned brown.

3. Drizzle oregano, lemon juice, and black pepper and serve.

Nutritional Fact:

- Total Time: 10 mins
- Serving: 2
- Calories 299 kcal
- Proteins 18 g
- Carbohydrates 3 g

- ➢ Cholesterol 64 g
- ➢ Fat 25 g

Ingredients:

- ➢ 1 tsp olive oil
- ➢ ¼ cup milk
- ➢ One sliced bell pepper (red)
- ➢ ½ salsa
- ➢ Two whole eggs
- ➢ One chopped white onion
- ➢ Four egg whites
- ➢ ½ tsp salt
- ➢ 1 tsp black pepper
- ➢ Pinch of cumin

Instructions:

1. heat olive oil on medium flame in a skillet, sauté onion, and red bell pepper for about five mins.

2. In a mixing bowl, whisk eggs, egg white, milk, salt, cumin, and black pepper.

3. In a baking dish, place a stir-fried onion mixture.

4. Add egg mixture over onion and bell pepper mixture.

5. place baking dish in a preheated oven at 350 degrees for 30 mins.

6. Make slices of the frittata and serve with salsa.

Nutritional Fact:

- ➢ Total Time: 50 mins

- ➢ Serving: 2
- ➢ Calories 202 kcal
- ➢ Proteins 17 g
- ➢ Carbohydrates 16 g
- ➢ Cholesterol 188 g
- ➢ Fat 8.5 g

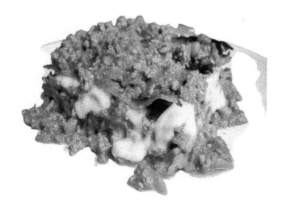

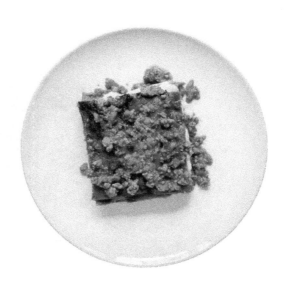

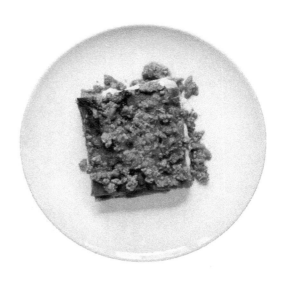

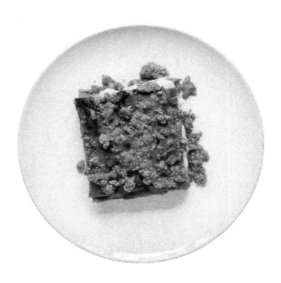

Ingredients:

- ➢ 4 ounces pancetta diced
- ➢ Five eggs
- ➢ 1/4 tsp salt to taste
- ➢ 1/2 cup chopped onion
- ➢ 1/2 tsp chopped garlic
- ➢ 1/2 cup chopped tomato
- ➢ 1/4 cup almond milk
- ➢ 1/2 cup chopped oregano
- ➢ 1/2 cup chopped basil
- ➢ 1 cup tomato sauce
- ➢ Black pepper to taste
- ➢ Red pepper flakes for garnishing
- ➢ 2/3 cup grated parmesan cheese
- ➢ Oregano for garnishing

Instructions:

1. In a pan, add onion and pancetta in a skillet and sauté for two mins.

2. Turn off the flame

3. In a mixing bowl, add cheese and milk and whisk them well.

4. Add tomato, herbs, garlic, tomato sauce, black pepper, salt, and mix.

5. Add tomato mixture in skillet with pancetta and onion.

6. Placing eggs in the pan makes a small space using a spatula by moving the mixture aside.

7. Break eggs and pour them in spaces created in a mixture: one egg in each space.

8. Put some cheese on the upper surface.

9. for 15 mins, bake in a preheated oven at 425 degrees

10. Use flakes and parsley to garnish and serve.

Nutritional Fact:

- ➢ Total Time: 28 mins
- ➢ Serving: 4
- ➢ Calories 207 kcal
- ➢ Proteins 14 g
- ➢ Carbohydrates 6 g
- ➢ Cholesterol 204 g
- ➢ Fat 14.4 g

47) Keto Stuffed Portobello Mushrooms

Ingredients:

- ➢ Four Portobello mushroom
- ➢ 1-ounce basil
- ➢ 4 ounces. cream cheese
- ➢ 1 tbsp Italian herb mixture
- ➢ Eight slices of provolone cheese
- ➢ 1 tsp salt
- ➢ 1 tsp minced garlic
- ➢ 1 tsp smoked paprika
- ➢ 24 ounces sliced black olives
- ➢ 1/2 tsp black pepper
- ➢ 1 tsp chopped onion

Instructions:

1. Whisk seasonings and cream cheese in a mixing bowl.

2. Pour cream cheese blend in a pan or small cups.

3. Place the second layer of one ounce of olives (sliced) on cream cheese mixture in cups.

4. Place the third layer of cheese.

5. Drizzle pepper or salt to enhance the flavor.

6. Cover the cups with foil.

7. Bake in a preheated oven at 425 degrees for 25 mins.

8. Garnish with basil leaves before serving.

Nutritional Fact:

- ➤ Total Time: 30 mins
- ➤ Serving: 4
- ➤ Calories 647 kcal
- ➤ Proteins 20 g
- ➤ Carbohydrates 5 g
- ➤ Cholesterol 30 g
- ➤ Fat 62 g

48) Keto broccoli cauliflower salad

Ingredients:

Amish salad

- ➤ ½ cup chopped onion
- ➤ 4 cup chopped broccoli and cauliflower stems and florets
- ➤ ¼ cup walnut
- ➤ Nine slices of chopped bacon

Amish dressing

- ➤ ½ tsp black pepper
- ➤ 1 cup mayonnaise
- ➤ tbsps sugar substitute
- ➤ ½ cup chopped onion
- ➤ 1 tsp salt
- ➤ 1 cup sour cream
- ➤ tbsp vinegar (apple cider)

Instructions:

1. Mix sweetener sour cream, onions, salt, mayonnaise, and pepper in a mixing bowl. The dressing is ready. Keep it aside.

2. In another bowl, mix broccoli and cauliflower and mix well.

3. Add dressing over the cauliflower mixture and toss to coat the vegetables with the dressing fully.

4. Add nuts and bacon and mix well.

5. It can store for three days in the refrigerator.

Nutritional Fact:

- ➤ Total Time: 25 mins
- ➤ Serving: 12
- ➤ Calories 118 kcal
- ➤ Proteins 4.2 g
- ➤ Carbohydrates 4.9 g
- ➤ Cholesterol 20 g
- ➤ Fat 9.1 g

49) Keto hamburger salad

Ingredients:

Sauce

- ➢ 1 tbsp chopped onions
- ➢ 3/4 cup Mayonnaise
- ➢ 1 tbsp vinegar
- ➢ 1/2 tsp paprika (smoked)
- ➢ 2tbsp Dill Pickles
- ➢ tsps swerve
- ➢ tsp Mustard

Salad

- ➢ 1 lb ground beef
- ➢ 1 cup cheddar cheese shredded
- ➢ 1 tsp kosher salt
- ➢ 4 cups lettuce chopped
- ➢ ½ cup onions sliced
- ➢ 1 tsp black pepper
- ➢ 1/4 cup dill pickles

Instructions:

1. First, prepare the dressing by combining mustard, paprika, mayonnaise, onion, pickles, swerve, and vinegar in a bowl. Set aside.

2. On medium flame, heat the pan, stir in ground beef and cook for 10 mins.

3. Sprinkle pepper and salt and cook until beef is done.

4. Mix onion, lettuce, cheese, and pickles in a bowl.

5. Add beef to the mixture and pour dressing over the beef. Toss well to mix everything thoroughly.

6. Serve.

Nutritional Fact:

➢ Total Time: 25 mins

➢ Serving: 4

➢ Calories 625 kcal

➢ Proteins 31 g

➢ Carbohydrates 5 g

➢ Cholesterol 0 g

➢ Fat 52 g

Conclusion

Accepting that the limitations of another eating routine can prove challenging at times, When it comes to food and plans often, they turn out to be so close to home and our families that it seems difficult to split away from them. Fortunately, there are simple approaches to make options in contrast to your number one food sources, so they fit inside keto, or if nothing else- stay inside a nearby window.

Assuming you do not experience any symptoms that come with medical conditions, a ketogenic diet can provide you with numerous advantages, particularly revolving around weight reduction. The main thing to retain is to eat an incredible equilibrium of vegetables, lean meat, and natural carbs.

In effect, adhering to the required nourishments is suggested to be the most proficient method for eating strongly, principally due to its simplicity and being a maintainable strategy. It is imperative to note that a great deal of exploration demonstrates that ketogenic slims down are hard to keep up with; Thus, the best yet effective solution is to locate a comfortable eating method that is suited to you. There are no stigmas around attempting new things, however, do not rush into it- take your time.

Ketones are at the focal point of the ketogenic diet- Your body produces ketones, a fuel particle, as an elective fuel source when the body lacks glucose. The process of delivering ketones happens when you decrease carbs and devour the perfect measure of protein.

When you have reached the point where you are eating keto compliant food products, your liver can convert muscle to fat ratio into ketones, where following this, it gets utilized as a fuel source by your body. At the point where the body is utilizing fat as a fuel source, you have entered ketosis. It permits the body to increase its rate of fat consumption significantly now and again. Furthermore, this helps with lessening pockets of undesirable fat. This fat consumption technique not exclusively helps you shed

211

lbs, but it can likewise avoid yearnings and forestall energy crashes for the day.

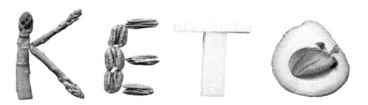

CPSIA information can be obtained
at www.ICGtesting.com
Printed in the USA
BVHW062008260221
601199BV00004B/177

9 781802 089851